A Woman's Book of YOGA

A Journal for Health and Self-Discovery

LOUISE TAYLOR

Charles E. Tuny, Inc.
Boston • Rutlana, Vermont • Tokyo

D1019661

Published in 1993 by
CHARLES E. TUTTLE COMPANY, INC.
of Rutland, Vermont, and Tokyo, Japan,
with editorial offices at 153 Milk Street,
Boston, Massachusetts 02109

Library of Congress Cataloging-in-Publication Data
Taylor, Louise.
A woman's book of yoga: a journal for health and self-discovery / by
Louise Taylor.
p. cm.
Includes bibliographical references.
ISBN 0-8048-1829-0
1. Yoga. I. Title.
RA781.7.T29 1993 93-21380
613.7'046'082--dc20 CIP

Design by Julie Gray, J. Campbell Design

Printed in the United States of America

Acknowledgments

With gratitude for all of her fantastic computer help, thanks to my daughter, Donna Taylor. I also want to thank all of my friends and associates at the Healing Arts Center, who have been so loving and caring.

Contents

Preface

As women, we are all seeking a way to achieve good health and inner peace in a world that is charged with tension and anxiety. Throughout my many years of taking and teaching yoga classes, I have found that the skills and understandings of this ancient tradition can be especially helpful in leading us to that goal.

I have also found that yoga is best learned in small increments, a little at a time. Seen as a gradual process, an unfolding, the stress of gaining immediate results is diminished and the learning process becomes an end in itself, providing an abundance of joyful self-discovery and new insights. For that reason I have chosen to present **A Woman's Book of Yoga** in a journal format because accomplishments derived from the study of yoga are very subtle and can be easily lost or not completely understood unless they are recorded for future comparison. Also, writing in a journal is an extremely useful tool because it will enable you to become aware of new accomplishments gained from each practice session.

All of the information that you will need for your study has been presented in a logical step-by-step progression of new ideas and concepts. Because the concepts are at first unfamiliar to those of us who are accustomed to living in a Western culture, I have designed this book to encourage you to interact with these new ideas in a way that will make them readily understandable and relevant to your daily life. If you use it as a journal and on a regular basis, it will become an aid to self-discovery by giving you a chance to pause and reflect on past experiences and future goals. It should be perceived as a constantly available source that you can use whenever you wish to record your many new experiences.

Willingness to participate fully in the study of yoga can also open channels of personal growth that lead to a sense of well-being on many different levels. Many yoga students gradually develop deeper understandings that allow them to become free of the negative demands of our competitive society. The values of harmony within nature and a sense of love and unity may slowly replace the desires for materialistic gain.

It is my hope that **A Woman's Book of Yoga** will afford you many hours of pleasure and become a source of inspiration to help you on your path of self-fulfillment and discovery.

Chapter 1

Origins of Yoga

❖

The Paths of Yoga

❖

How Yoga Can Benefit You

❖

Getting Started

❖

Helpful Knowledge for
Hatha Yoga Practice

❖

Your Journal

Origins of Yoga

Yoga originated in ancient India. Begun by Tibetan monks more than six thousand years ago, the techniques and theories were initially handed down orally by a chain of teachers and students. At first its teachings were secret, as were those of its offshoots, among them karate and t'ai chi. The first written account of yoga is attributed to the Indian sage Patanjali, who codified the complete system in the second century B.C. His **Yoga Sutras** remain one of India's most important writings.

The word yoga is derived from the ancient Sanskrit root verb **yuj**, which means "to join" or "unite." It signifies the union of the conscious mind with the deeper levels of the unconscious or universal mind, which ultimately results in a totally integrated personality. The yogic ideal of unification is called **mukusha** and connotes a perfect balance or state of naturalness. The philosophy stresses that the whole of life strives toward this ideal, which is described by the Christian religion as the peace that passeth all understanding. Yoga teaches that when we begin to search for balance and natural harmony in our lives, we begin to grow on a path that leads to deeper understanding and fulfillment. At such a time we learn that satisfaction comes from something we find deep within, and does not rely on external stimulation.

In the sixth chapter of the **Bhagavad Gita**, which is the most important authority on yoga philosophy, Krishna explains to Arjuna the meaning of yoga as a deliverance from the sorrows of this world.

The Eight Limbs of Yoga

The first Western travelers in the East, in the times of Marco Polo, returned with stories of philosophers and sages who were described as being utterly serene, detached, and apparently unaffected by the ordinary difficulties of living. They were indifferent to pain and were able to control their minds and bodies in ways that, to Western observers, seemed miraculous. These sages were Hindu yogis. In the **Yoga Sutras**, Patanjuli outlined in detail the physical and mental achievements necessary for one aspiring to this state. The book contains one hundred and ninety-six short aphorisms that describe the philosophy of yoga and the means of making it a viable reality in the life of a yogi (a yogi is a follower of yoga). Patanjali divided his work into four chapters. In the second chapter he describes the eight limbs of yoga, which provide the core of yogic philosophy:

Yama: abstention from evil.

Niyamas: observances.

Asanas: postures. Out of the thousands of postures then in use, Patanjali chose eighty-four. In India today these same postures are basic to the s t u d y of yoga.

Pranayama: breath control.

Dharana: concentration.

Dhyana: meditation.

Pratyahara: sense withdrawal.

Samadhi: self-realization.

Of these, **yamas** and **niyamas** should be examined more closely because they describe rules of moral conduct that are required of the student of yoga. **Niyamas** are the rules of conduct that apply to individual discipline, whereas **yamas** are universal in their application. The five abstinences or **yamas** are as follows:

Ahimsa: nonviolence: Mahatma Gandhi, one of the most revered philosophers and statesmen of India, founded his philosophy on **ahimsa** and **satya** (truth). He believed that these represent the soul force (**Satyagraha**), which he felt to be vastly superior to brute force represented by bombs and guns. He stated repeatedly that soul force is indispensible in transforming the politics of bloodshed into the politics of human welfare and world peace.

Satya: truthfulness.

Asteya: nonstealing.

Brahmacharya: continence of the body, speech, and mind (this can also be translated as chastity or fidelity).

Aparigrapha: simplification of life by not hoarding or collecting possessions.

The following are the five observances or **niyamas**:

Saucha: purity.

Santosa: contentment.

Tapas: austerity.

Svadhyaya: study.

Ishvara pranidhana: worship of God or the universal soul. By understanding the eight limbs of yoga we can see that practitioners are provided with a complete philosophy that gives them an intellectual understanding of the nature of creation, the nature of humans, and the relationship between them.

The Paths of Yoga

The schools or paths of yoga are numerous. Each student is generally attracted to the particular form which best answers his or her own needs. In many ways, the differences are largely a matter of emphasis because many of the paths overlap to some extent. Each one leads to personal development and eventually to a state of higher consciousness where the individual self merges with the universal self, bringing people and nature into complete harmony. Many serious students choose more than one path. Swami Vivekananda, who was instrumental in introducing yoga to the United States around the turn of the century, believed in a synthesis of the various yogas to achieve self-realization. Others believe that it is more beneficial to follow one path to their goal.

Hatha Yoga

Although necessary to all existence, balance is often upset. Yoga attempts to restore it through a threefold path of development—physical, mental, and spiritual. Yoga claims that there is no artificial separation between that which is body and that which is mind. This is the logic behind the fact that all yoga instruction begins with the physical, with hatha yoga, the philosophy of physical well-being. The goal is to gain control of the body's energy flow and to direct it in positive, healing ways. The vital energy called **chi** by the Chinese and **ki** by the Japanese is called **prana** in India. **Prana** is everywhere and in everything; it is the basic force that animates all matter. In the study of yoga the life force or **prana** is closely associated with breathing practices that control and direct this important energy. Freed and able to flow throughout the body, it can stimulate both body and mind; blocked and distorted, it can sap and deplete our vitality.

The postures and breathing techniques of hatha yoga combine to provide vibrant energy and well-being. Each posture is enhanced by the addition of proper breathing (**pranayama**). The stretches, breathing, and deep relaxation exercises of hatha yoga balance and tone the entire body. They provide an effective method for dealing with our normal fast-paced lives, and give quick, observable results in relieving stress and tension.

The name hatha is made up of two Sanskrit roots: **ha**, which stands for the sun, and **tha** for the moon. In the science of hatha yoga, the right side of the body is the positive, male, sun, heat side, the left side is the negative, female, moon, cool side. Through the practice of hatha yoga the two sides and their characteristic forces are brought into balance. Thus one can obtain physical health, mental clarity, and steady strength of mind and character. The practice and eventual mastery of the postures and breathing patterns result in a balanced and steady mind and body.

Hatha yoga asanas (bench or steady positions) are designed to give maximum flexibility and strength to the skeletal, muscular, and nervous systems. They stretch and strengthen the spine and work, with the aid of breathing exercises, to balance and revitalize the body. While doing the stretches the vital organs are massaged and blood circulation is increased. The asanas are practiced not only to achieve a state of well-being but as a preparation for meditation. To meditate effectively, it is important to have a strong, flexible body that is able to remain in a meditative posture for long periods without becoming fatigued.

You will notice that the asanas are named for animals and natural phenomena. The reason for this can be found in the **Vedas**, ancient Hindu scriptures, which describe how yoga exercises were created and designed by the king of yogis, Lord Shiva, at the beginning of time. Lord Shiva observed how animals remained strong and healthy in harsh and varied environments. After studying their breathing and sleeping patterns as well as their movements, he isolated the underlying techniques that enabled them to survive efficiently and, from them, developed the hatha yoga system.

Hatha yoga is presented in fuller detail because it is the main subject of this book. However, it is useful and interesting to gain an overview of the entire yogic system.

Mantra Yoga

A mantra is a repeated phrase. **Japa** is the term used to describe the actual repetition. Therefore, mantra yoga is sometimes called **japa** yoga. Followers of mantra yoga repeat certain mantras thousands of times. A mantra takes the place of usual thought patterns and focuses the mind on the vibration of the mantra. The mantra and its goal merge and become one and the same.

Bhakti Yoga

Bhakti yoga involves concentration and meditation on the divine. It is the yoga of faith, devotion, and worship. People engaged in appreciating art, music, or nature practice **bhakti** yoga whether or not they call it by that name. Service toward humanity and animals and an unselfish striving to see the universal principle in all things is the path of one practicing this yoga. **Bhakti** yoga is often combined with mantra yoga. Chanting the mantra with love, the yogi becomes inspired and filled with bliss.

Karma Yoga

This is the yoga of action. Its name comes from the Sanskrit **kri**, which means "to do." It is based on the law of cause and effect, with good deeds producing good results. Followers of karma yoga feel that they are a necessary unit in the whole process of life.

Jnana Yoga

In Sanskrit **jnana** means "to know." This is the path of knowledge or intellectual attainment. The truths of existence and the nature of the self are examined. In this yoga students focus on themselves, not as the body, feelings, personality, or intellect, but as their user. This yoga raises the seeker above limitations and attempts to recognize the similarities and truths in all philosophies.

Raja Yoga

Raja signifies royal, or kingly. This is the yoga of self-mastery through mental control. It seeks to gain control over the stream of thoughts, attempting to check that flow and still the mind by means of concentration (**dharana**) and contemplation (**dhyana**). By these practices a state of superconsciousness (**samadhi**) may be reached. Raja yoga is closely linked with hatha yoga and the two are often practiced together. Hatha yoga aims at mastering the body and raja yoga aims at mastering the mind.

Laya Yoga

This term, meaning "latency" in the sense of hidden, defines a type of yoga applied to stilling the mind in order to awaken and direct the inner force called **kundalini**. The **kundalini** is seen as a life force that purifies the body by traveling through each of the energy centers (**chakras**).

How Yoga Can Benefit You

The following benefits have often been recorded by women who regularly practice yoga at least three times a week: weight loss; relief from such conditions as insomnia, headache, backache, constipation, sinusitis, and asthma; improved balance and posture; improved concentration; increased strength and flexibility; reduced mental strain, stress, and tension; improved relaxation; improved circulation and breathing; and improved condition of skin, eyes, and hair. These and many other positive changes occur through a regular commitment to practice yoga because it is a complete program that involves the entire individual physically, mentally, and spiritually. A basic premise is that a definite link exists between mind and body, that whatever affects one affects the other.

One of the most rewarding aspects of yoga practice is discovering how mind and body can unite in a harmony of movement and coordination. You will open to new vistas of understanding about yourself. While participating in many other forms of exercise it is possible to allow your mind to wander. In yoga, your mental focus on the stretch, coordinated with deep and regular breathing, produces an internal and external unity that gradually increases with practice. This concentration eventually becomes a form of mental discipline that you can apply to all phases of your life.

Yoga is extremely beneficial for anyone of any age. With continued practice of this versatile system of exercise, you can see results quickly because, as you release tensions, you liberate vast resources of energy.

Practicing yoga also promotes a high level of organic health. It can help you to keep a youthful bearing and outlook which radiate feelings that every woman wants, energy, beauty, and poise.

Yoga increases circulation and flexibility. Your spine provides the housing for the central and autonomic nervous systems, and thus your entire body benefits as your spine becomes more flexible. Movement can become a pleasure as your joints begin to function with greater ease, and your muscles start to work more smoothly and efficiently.

Many women are first drawn to yoga as a way to keep fit and supple. Others come seeking relief for a specific complaint. Whatever your reason, it can become an important part of your life as an instrument for your well-being and self-discovery.

Getting Started

It is helpful to set aside a specific time each day to work with this book. You will need at least a half hour when you know that you will not be disturbed. If you practice in the morning, you will not be as limber as you are later in the day. The morning stretches, however, will help you to prepare for the day ahead. If you practice in the evening, the stretches will relax you for a good night's sleep.

Set aside a place for your practice that is clean and pleasant. It should be well ventilated but not drafty. The room temperature should be warm enough to allow you to exercise comfortably. You will need adequate space in which to stretch fully, and a carpet or a rug to protect you from the hardness of the floor. Do not use a spongy or air-filled mattress, though, because soft surfaces do not support your spine.

Be sure you will not be distracted. Turn off the television, radio, and, if possible, the telephone during the time you have designated for your practice.

You do not have to purchase special clothing, but be sure that what you wear is clean, light, and comfortable. Remove your wristwatch and any loose jewelry such as earrings, bracelets, and necklaces that might distract you.

Wait at least an hour after eating and, if possible, empty your bladder and bowels before you start.

Wherever necessary, limitations are included with the asana instructions. Consult the specific directions for each posture before you start your program. If you have any physical problems that warrant attention, check with your physician before you begin.

Helpful Knowledge for
Hatha Yoga Practice

Always use caution and common sense when practicing yoga postures. Move slowly and smoothly in and out of each asana, without bouncing or stretching to the point of strain. The number of repetitions given for each posture are to be used as a guideline only. Your body will know how long you should hold each one and how many repetitions you should do.

If you do not feel comfortable with an asana, such as the wheel, or head stand, hold off doing it until you are ready to add it to your program.

Do each asana with full awareness and concentration, having read all of the directions and limitations on each page. Always concentrate on your breathing while practicing the exercises. Inhale and exhale through the nose. As you breathe in, feel your body filling with energy. Imagine that you are sending energy to the muscles you are stretching.

You will notice that, except for Chapter 2 (warm-ups) and Chapter 15, each chapter contains two asanas for you to practice.

Learn them in the sequence presented, adding two at a time to your program. By the time you complete Chapter 14, you will be able to do an entire program of yoga postures. Chapter 15 contains balance postures to challenge you further. It would be best to attempt these postures after you have taken the time to strengthen your body with the basic asanas.

When you start your program, always warm up with the sun salutation, head rolls, shoulder rotations, foot-limbering exercises, and the back stretch. Add the spinal rock and the butterfly to your warm-ups as time allows. During practice, choose at least one or two of the breathing exercises found in Chapter 3, and conclude each of your practice sessions with at least five minutes of complete rest in **shavasana**.

Your Journal

A journal is a way of keeping track of your pathway to success. It encourages you and points out how well you are doing. Here are some suggestions to help you to use your journal effectively.

In your journal, record your reactions to the asanas. Take a few minutes to do this each time you practice, especially in the beginning when you are learning to do the exercises. At the end of Chapter 15 you will find additional pages that will enable you to continue to record your progress.

Every asana is accompanied by a progress chart on which to record the degree of ease or difficulty you encounter in each posture. As you continue to record your entries, you will soon be able to observe many new and rewarding changes.

Each chapter contains two special sections: New Understandings and Insights. The New Understandings have been included to allow you to gain a greater appreciation for the many aspects of yoga. The section on Insights will enable you to become more aware of your environment, your physical body, your mind, and your spirit. First complete the asanas in your daily program, and then take a few moments to thoughtfully and carefully work the other sections of your journal.

Chapter 2

New Understandings:
The Importance of Stretching and
Flexibility

Warm-ups
Sun Salutation (**Surya Namaskar**)
Head Rolls
Shoulder Rotations
Foot-Limbering Exercises
Shoulder Clasp (**Veerasana**)
Spinal Rock
The Butterfly (**Bhadrasana**)
Pose of a Child (**Balasana**)
Corpse Pose (**Shavasana**)

Insight:
Discovering New Words and Ideas

New Understandings
The Importance of Stretching and Flexibility

We can learn a great deal about stretching by watching cats or dogs. They instinctively know how to stretch. They do it spontaneously, never over-stretching, continually and naturally tuning their muscles. By regularly practicing the yoga postures, you will begin to experience a sense of balance and inner harmony as your spine and muscles become more supple.

It is interesting to note that flexibility can be improved more quickly and retained longer than any other aspect of physical fitness. Regular practice of yoga postures will increase your range of motion by allowing you to move freely and efficiently with minimal resistance. The asanas can prevent joint stiffening and muscle shortening that often accompany injury, inactivity, and aging. As you stretch various parts of your body, you begin to focus on them and get in touch with them in a new and meaningful way. Stretching also helps loosen the mind's control so that your body can experience movement for its own sake and pleasure.

A limber spine and a young body go together. Those who have retained the elasticity of their spines and limbs appear youthful and alive. When your spine is flexible and in alignment, the result can be seen in your whole body, in the way it moves and functions. The well-being of your spinal column has a direct effect on your health and vitality because that structure is the foundation of your body. The thirty-three vertebrae enclose the spinal cord, which is made up of all of the nerves that stem from your brain. Each vertebra has openings through which the branches of the nerves spread out, going to every part of your body.

When your spine is healthy and limber, the vertebrae and nerves function properly. When a vertebra is out of alignment, however, it affects the nerves, muscles and internal organs associated with it. Also, muscular tension tends to collect around any imbalanced area, ultimately causing back pain.

During yoga practice you will stretch your spine in all six possible directions: forward, backward, bending to each side, and twisting to each side. This creates a balance and symmetry in your spinal column which you can enhance after you have learned all of the asanas by choosing complementary sets of postures. For example, the plow pose curves your spine forward and the cobra pose curves it backward. Each time you bend in one direction you can choose a second posture that curves in the opposite direction. This will promote the health of your entire spine, from the cervical vertebrae in your neck to the lowest of the lumbar vertebrae.

Not only do the asanas promote physical balance and harmony, they also feel good when practiced correctly. They are peaceful and relaxing. As you stretch you should just go only as far as you comfortably can, regardless of where it may be. As you hold each stretch you will gradually impart increasing elasticity to your muscles, joints, and spine. This occurs regardless of your age or current physical condition. Once achieved, you will find that you can retain this wonderfully flexible state for your entire lifetime.

Warm-ups

Before you begin to do the asanas, prepare your body gradually with a series of warm-up exercises. These will loosen the muscles and ease stiffness from your joints. It is extremely important to warm up from head to toe. Always begin with the sun salutation, and include head and shoulder rotations, foot-limbering exercises, and heel raises. As time allows, you can choose one or two of the other exercises presented in this chapter.

Surya Namaskar or salutation to the sun, is a graceful series of movements that are very helpful in preparing you for the more difficult asanas by stretching your entire body. As you synchronize the movements with your breathing, you also develop coordination and breath control. If you do not have time to do a complete yoga program, you can derive great benefit by doing the sun salutation.

This exercise can be extremely helpful in energizing and stimulating your mind and body when you first get up in the morning. The sun salutation can be practiced rapidly and will have an immediate aerobic effect. Performed slowly, it releases tension in your muscles and removes fatigue. Like all strenuous asanas, it should be followed by a few minutes of complete relaxation. Initially, the movements should be performed slowly and gracefully as you perfect each posture. In combining breathing with the movements, always inhale when you stretch upward and exhale when bending forward. Once you have learned the sequence of each asana, you can allow your own breathing and body response to determine your rate of movement.

Sun Salutation
(Surya Namaskar)

The twelve positions of this exercise
should be done slowly and rhythmically.

Position 1. Prayer pose
(pranamasana)
Exhale. Stand straight.
Place your palms together in front of
your chest.
Relax your body.

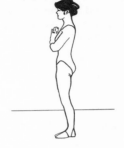

Position 2. Raised-arms pose
(hasta uttanasana)
Inhale. Stretch your arms above your
head, keeping them a shoulder-width
apart.
Bend backward as far as you can.

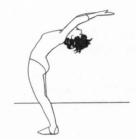

Position 3. Hand-to-foot pose
(padahastasana)
Exhale. Stretch forward until your hands
are in line with your feet.
Bring your forehead close to your knees
and keep your legs as straight as possible.

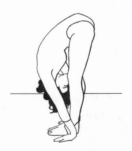

CHART YOUR PROGRESS - Degree of difficulty

	Hard							Easy		Hard							Easy
Date	1	2	3	4	5	6	7	8	Date	1	2	3	4	5	6	7	8
5/9 X																	

Position 4. Equestrian pose (ashwa sanchalanasana)

Inhale. With a backward step, stretch your right leg away from your body with your knee touching the floor. Keep the palms of your hands beside your left foot. Arch your back and look up.

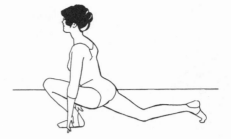

Position 5. Quadruped pose. (catuspadasana)

Exhale. Hold your breath out, and move your left leg back so that you are resting on your hands and toes in a push-up position. Keep your back and head straight.

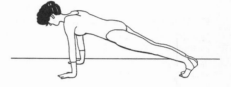

Position 6. Salute with eight limbs (ashtanga namaskara)

Inhale. As you exhale, lower your body to the floor keeping your hips and abdomen raised. Your toes, knees, hands, and chest should touch the floor.

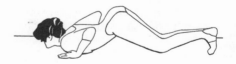

Position 7. Serpent pose (bhujangasana)

Inhale. Straighten your arms as you raise your upper body from the waist. Bend backward as far as you can, looking up and back.

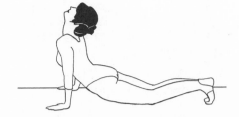

Position 8. The Mountain pose (parvatasana)

Exhale. Turn your toes forward so that your feet are flat on the floor.
Lift your body up to form a triangle.
Keep your head down and your arms and legs straight.

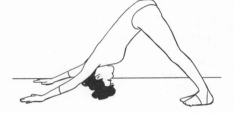

Position 9. Equestrian pose (ashwa sanvhalanasana)

Inhale. Bring your right foot forward next to your hands, and at the same time, lower your left knee to the floor.
Arch your back and look up.

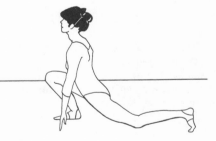

Position 10. Hand-to-foot pose (padahastasana)

Exhale.

Bring your left leg forward, keeping your knees straight and your hands beside your feet.

Lower your head down to your knees.

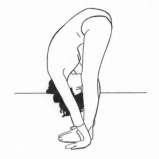

Position 11. Raised-arm pose (hasta uttanasana)

Inhale. Stretch your arms over your head. Bend as far backward as you comfortably can.

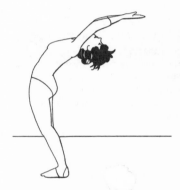

Position 12. Prayer pose (pranamasana)

Exhale. Return to your starting position and start the sequence again, using your left leg as the leading leg.

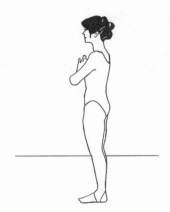

Chart Your Progress
Body Awareness

Sun Salutation

Date

Head Rolls

Benefits
Loosens and relieves tension in the neck.

Basic position
Sit cross-legged or in a half-lotus position with your hands on your knees.

Instructions
Slowly rotate your head five times in a large circle clockwise. Change to a counterclockwise direction and repeat five more times.

Breathing
Inhale and exhale slowly as you rotate your head.

Limitation
Avoid rotating your head backward, as this may cause unnecessary neck tension or strain. Your head rotations should be limited to each side and forward.

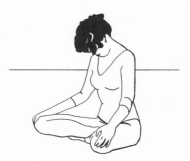

Position 1

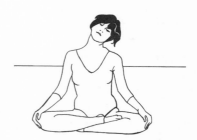

Position 2

CHART YOUR PROGRESS - Degree of difficulty

	Hard							Easy		Hard							Easy
Date	1	2	3	4	5	6	7	8	Date	1	2	3	4	5	6	7	8

Chart Your Progress
Body Awareness

Head Rolls

Date

_____

_____

_____

_____

_____

_____

_____

_____

_____

_____

_____

_____

_____

_____

_____

_____

_____

_____

Shoulder Rotations

Benefits
Loosens the shoulder joints, and relieves tension in the shoulders and upper back.

Basic position
Sit cross-legged or in a half-lotus position with your hands on your knees.

Instructions
Slowly rotate your shoulders in a large circle. Repeat five times forward. Change direction and repeat five more times.

Breathing
Inhale slowly while raising your shoulders. Exhale slowly as your shoulders come down.

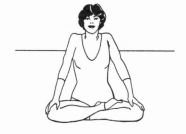

CHART YOUR PROGRESS - Degree of difficulty																
	Hard						Easy			Hard						Easy
Date	1	2	3	4	5	6	7	8	Date	1	2	3	4	5	6	7	8

Chart Your Progress
Body Awareness

Shoulder Rotations

Date

Foot-Limbering Exercises

Benefits
Loosens the joints in the feet.

Basic position
Sit straight with your legs outstretched. Your hands may be placed on your thighs or behind you for balance.

Instructions
Flex and point your feet ten times, then alternate for ten times with one foot flexing and the other pointing. Next, rotate your feet in opposite circles ten times.

Breathing
Breathe fully and slowly, and send the energy of your breath to your feet.

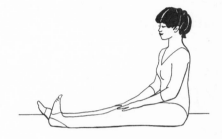

CHART YOUR PROGRESS - Degree of difficulty																	
	Hard							Easy		Hard							Easy
Date	1	2	3	4	5	6	7	8	Date	1	2	3	4	5	6	7	8

Chart Your Progress
Body Awareness

Foot-Limbering Exercises

Date

_____

_____

_____

_____

_____

_____

_____

_____

_____

_____

_____

_____

_____

_____

_____

_____

Shoulder Clasp
(Veerasana)

Benefits
Strengthens and stretches the back, and strengthens the arms and shoulders.

Basic position
Sit on the floor cross-legged or in a half-lotus posture, arms comfortably at your side.

Instructions
Bend your left elbow and place your left hand behind your back.
Reach over your right shoulder with your right hand and interlace your fingers.
Slowly bend forward as far as you can without straining.
Briefly hold the posture.
Slowly return to the basic position.
Change arms and repeat on the other side.
Repeat three times on each side.

Breathing
Inhale in the basic position.
Exhale as you stretch forward.
Breathe normally in the stretch.
Exhale as you return to the basic position.

Limitation
At first your hands may not come together easily or at all. If this is the case, place your hands in the above position but allow a space between your hands. You will probably find that one side is easier to do than the other. As you develop more flexibility and strength, both sides will become better aligned.

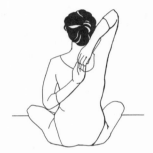

Position 1

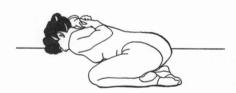

Position 2

CHART YOUR PROGRESS - Degree of difficulty																	
	Hard						Easy			Hard							Easy
Date	1	2	3	4	5	6	7	8	Date	1	2	3	4	5	6	7	8

Chart Your Progress
Body Awareness
Shoulder Clasp

Date

_____

_____

_____

_____

_____

_____

_____

_____

_____

_____

_____

_____

_____

_____

_____

_____

_____

_____

_____

Spinal Rock

Benefits
Warms up your muscles, limbers the spine, and inverts blood flow; excellent toning for the entire body.

Basic position
Sit on the floor.
Clasp your arms around your knees, or sit cross-legged and hold on to your feet.

Instructions
Be sure your knees remain bent throughout the exercise.
Holding your initial position, roll backward on your back as far as you comfortably can.
Keep your chin tucked toward your chest and your back slightly rounded.
Maintaining your momentum, roll forward to a seated position.
Repeat five to seven times, maintaining a gentle rocking motion.

Breathing
Inhale in the basic position.
Exhale while rocking backward.
Inhale while rocking forward.

Limitations
Do not do this asana if you have spinal problems or are menstruating heavily.

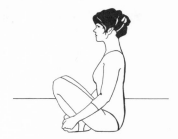

Position 1

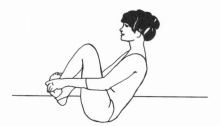

Position 2

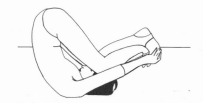

Position 3

CHART YOUR PROGRESS - Degree of difficulty																	
	Hard						Easy			Hard							Easy
Date	1	2	3	4	5	6	7	8	Date	1	2	3	4	5	6	7	8

Chart Your Progress
Body Awareness

Spinal Rock

Date
_____

_____

_____

_____

_____

_____

_____

_____

_____

_____

_____

_____

_____

_____

_____

_____

_____

_____

_____

_____

Butterfly Pose
(Bhadrasana)

Benefits
Stretches hip, knee, and ankle joints, and strengthens back and abdominal muscles. Preparation for the half-lotus posture.

Basic position
Sit with your legs outstretched.
Bring the soles of your feet together, pulling them as close as possible to the body.
Keep your back straight.

Instructions
Grasp your toes with both hands.
Gently try to press your knees close to the floor.
Continue sitting with your back as straight as possible.
Slowly and rhythmically repeat the action ten times.

Breathing
Breathe normally.

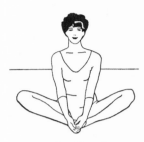

Position 1

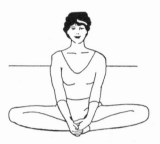

Position 2

CHART YOUR PROGRESS - Degree of difficulty																
	Hard						Easy			Hard						Easy
Date	1	2	3	4	5	6	7	8	Date	1	2	3	4	5	6	7	8

Chart Your Progress
Body Awareness

Butterfly Pose

Date

_____

_____

_____

_____

_____

_____

_____

_____

_____

_____

_____

_____

_____

_____

_____

_____

_____

Pose of a Child
(Balasana)

This is an excellent preparation for the more difficult postures. Be sure that your breathing is slow and comfortable.

Benefits
Massages the abdominal organs, and separates the vertebrae slightly, which allows
the spinal nerves to be stretched and
toned gently.
It is an excellent relaxation posture.

Instructions
Relax your whole body and close your
eyes.
Drop your forehead to the floor and
relax all the muscles in your neck, back,
and stomach.
Relax your arms and legs.
Remain in the posture for two or three
minutes.
Slowly return to the basic position.
Repeat during your practice whenever
you wish.

Breathing
Exhale slowly while bending forward.
Breathe deeply while in the posture.
Inhale as you return to the basic position.

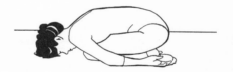

CHART YOUR PROGRESS - Degree of difficulty																
	Hard							Easy		Hard						Easy
Date	1	2	3	4	5	6	7	8	Date	1	2	3	4	5	6	7	8

Chart Your Progress
Body Awareness

Pose of a Child

Date

_____

_____

_____

_____

_____

_____

_____

_____

_____

_____

_____

_____

_____

_____

_____

_____

_____

Corpse Pose
(Shavasana)

By taking a minute or two to relax, after completing the desired number of repetitions for each asana, you will allow your body to absorb the maximum benefit from each stretch. You should also conclude your practice with three to five minutes of **shavasana** each time you practice yoga.

Benefits
Relaxes your entire body, especially when combined with deep breathing.

Basic position
Lie flat on your back with your arms beside your body, palms facing upward. Move your feet slightly apart to a comfortable position and close your eyes.

Instructions
Relax your whole body.

Breathing
Concentrate on your breath and let it become rhythmic and natural.
Become aware of the inhalation and exhalation.
If your mind starts to wander, bring it back to the breath.
By focusing your mind on your breath for just a few minutes, a state of deep relaxation will occur.

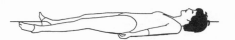

CHART YOUR PROGRESS - Degree of difficulty

Date	Hard 1	2	3	4	5	6	7	Easy 8	Date	Hard 1	2	3	4	5	6	7	Easy 8

Chart Your Progress
Body Awareness

Corpse Pose

Date

_____

_____

_____

_____

_____

_____

_____

_____

_____

_____

_____

_____

_____

_____

_____

_____

_____

_____

Insight
Discovering New Words and Ideas

As you progress through your journal you will discover many words that are new to you and many new ideas that are of interest. It will help you to remember the new words and concepts if you use this page to write them down when you discover them. Your understanding of the complete yoga will grow immensely as you establish the habit of recording your new knowledge.

Chapter 3

New Understandings:
Yogic Breathing (**Pranayama**)

Asanas
Double Angle Pose (**Dwi Konasana**)
The Fish (**Matsyasana**)

Insight:
Coordinating Your Mind and Body in
Harmony

New Understandings

Yogic Breathing

(Pranayama)

In Sanskrit, **prana** is defined as "the life force" or "vital energy." **Ayama** is translated as "to pause" or "to control." **Pranayama**, or yogic breathing, influences the flow of **prana** in the **nadis** (pranic or vital energy channels) that are related to the nervous system. Since respiration affects the heart, slow, relaxed breathing will slow the heart rate and faster breaths will accelerate it.

Breathing changes according to circumstances. When a person is angry or upset the rate and force of the breath increases. A calm person will take slower breaths and feel at ease. While thinking, we usually breathe through the left nostril with a greater flow of air. The breath flowing more fully through the right nostril is associated with physical action. As our activities fluctuate, the change in nostril breathing alternates. Exhalation predominates during sleep and brings rest. Inhalation predominates during our waking hours and is influenced by our moods and the external environment. **Pranayama** ensures that the flow of **prana** throughout the body is free and unimpeded. To gain mastery of the body and mind, it is first necessary to understand how breathing influences bodily changes.

To maintain a state of balance, breathing should always be rhythmic and harmonious. Most people breathe incorrectly, using only a small portion of their normal lung capacity. Shallow respiration leaves stagnant air in the lower regions of the lungs. By breathing incorrectly we often bring ill health to our bodies, which is unnecessary, considering the plentiful supply of oxygen. By learning to breathe correctly we can begin to experience an increase in health and energy.

Abdominal or Diaphragmatic Breathing

The diaphragm is a strong muscle membrane that separates the lungs from the abdominal organs. The lower it moves during inhalation, the more air is inhaled into the lungs. To experience this breath, sit straight or lie flat on your back and place one hand on your navel. As you inhale deeply your hand will rise as your abdomen expands. As you exhale deeply notice how your hand moves down as your abdomen contracts. Maximum expulsion of air from the lungs occurs when the contraction of the abdomen is accentuated.

Thoracic or Chest Breathing

The breath moves the rib cage outward and upward during inhalation.

When you exhale, your ribs move inward and downward.

The combination of abdominal and chest breathing allows you to inhale the optimum amount of air and to exhale the maximum amount of stale air.

Your daily practice should always include one of the following breathing exercises. As you practice them, you will experience the many beneficial ways yogic breathing can improve your health and vitality, and begin to experience a heightened sense of well-being. Try to practice **pranayama** several additional times a day, choosing the technique that is appropriate to your needs.

The Complete Breath

This exercise increases your lung capacity. It helps to cleanse your blood, and expands your chest cavity, allowing all parts of your lungs to be filled with oxygen. You may stand, sit, or lie on your back to do the exercise.

Focus on a steady and continuous flow of air from the lowest to the highest portion of your lungs. Breathe continuously and as slowly as possible.

Inhale and fill the lower part of your lungs (your abdomen should expand gently).

Continue inhaling and fill the upper portion of your lungs by expanding the upper part of your chest (your chest will rise slowly).

To fill the uppermost part of your lungs, slightly draw in your lower abdomen.

At the end of your inhalation, occasionally raise your shoulders to permit the air to enter the upper lobes of your lungs.

Retain your breath for as long as you comfortably can.

Exhale slowly and contract your abdomen slightly. When the air is completely exhaled, relax your chest and abdomen.

Practice this exercise frequently, and do it whenever you become tense and tired. Your inhalations and exhalations should be done very slowly to allow ample time to complete each step. With just a few days of practice you will begin to find that the complete breath revitalizes and cleanses your body, and brings about a deep sense of peace.

The Complete Breath Variation

Lie on your back with your arms by your sides. Practice the same inhalation as before, and with it, raise your arms overhead until the back of your hands touch the floor. As you slowly release the air, bring your arms forward and down to your sides. Repeat three times.

The Cleansing Breath

The cleansing breath is especially beneficial before a meal and whenever you feel fatigued. It clears the sinuses and respiratory system.

Exhale as deeply and as vigorously as possible.

Take a deep breath.

Exhale immediately through the nose as you contract your abdomen.

Repeat at least five times. Resume normal breathing.

Alternate Nostril Breathing

This exercise cleanses the nasal passages and has a calming effect. Sit with your back straight.

With your right thumb, gently apply an upward pressure to the bone of your right nostril. Inhale deeply and smoothly through your left nostril.

Retain the air for a few seconds.

Close your left nostril with your ring finger and gently press upward into the bone.

Release your thumb and slowly exhale through the right nostril until all of the air is expelled.

Leave your ring finger on your left nostril and inhale in the same way through your right nostril.

Close the right nostril with your thumb and exhale through your left nostril.

Repeat this breath slowly at least five times.

Your breath should be even and under control. After you have practiced the exercise, try to add counting. Inhale to the count of six and exhale to the count of twelve. The long exhalations have a deeply calming effect.

The Ha Breath

This is a revitalizing breath that will enable you to refresh and recharge your body at any time.

Stand with your legs apart.

Inhale deeply, raising your arms up from each side until they are stretched above your head.

Throw the upper half of your body forward, bending from the waist, at the same time letting your arms fall forward and expelling the breath with a strong blast, making the sound "ha."

Let your body hang loosely from the waist, arms swinging, head hanging as you repeat the ha sound several times.

Stand up slowly and repeat two more times.

The Bellows Breath (Bastrika)

This exercise imitates the action of a blacksmith's bellows. Emphasis is on a forceful expulsion of breath through the nose. Its rhythm is deep, quick, and vigorous. It helps to cleanse the bloodstream.

Lie on your back with your arms at your sides, or sit with your back completely straight.

Inhale fully.

Exhale forcefully through the nose, at the same time contract the abdomen and expel air with a powerful push from the diaphragm and thrust from the throat.

When you release the contraction, your lungs will automatically take in air.

Gradually build up to ten rapid expulsions; after your last one, inhale deeply to fill your lungs with air, exhale slowly, and relax.

Invigorating Pranayama

There is a cycle of breathing exercises for invigorating your entire system. They are done in a standing position and are designed to expel all of the stale air in your lungs. Do each one two times, concentrating on your breath. Once you have memorized the sequence you will have a powerful tool to use whenever you feel fatigued.

Inhale and raise your arms forward, parallel with the floor.

Grasp an imaginary stick, and hold your breath for six counts.

Exhale and lower your arms.

Inhale as completely as possible.

Retain the breath and tense every muscle of your body.

Exhale and relax.

Inhale and rise up onto the tips of your toes.

Retain the breath as long as you comfortably can.

Exhale and return to a normal standing position.

Inhale and raise both arms above your head, putting your palms together.

Hold your breath for six counts.

Exhale and lower your arms.

Inhale and rise up onto your toes, raise your arms above your head.

Palms together.

Hold your breath for six counts.

As you exhale slowly lower your arms and consciously relax your legs and feet.

Relaxing **Pranayama**

The following exercises can be used to bring about a state of calmness and relaxation.

The Waterfall

This exercise will enable you to relax deeply.

Inhale deeply.

Retain your breath briefly.

Exhale through slightly parted lips for as long as you can.

Repeat as often as you wish.

Cooling Breath

This exercise induces muscular relaxation and quenches thirst.

Sit with your back straight.

Fold your tongue into a trough and extend it beyond your lips.

Inhale slowly and deeply through the folded tongue.

Retain the breath as long as you comfortably can.

Exhale through the nose.

Droning Breath

When the breath is slowly released, with a controlled humming sound, the resonance is felt in the upper nasal passages between the eyebrows. This will enable you to relax and to concentrate more clearly.

Inhale deeply.

Hum as you exhale through the mouth with your lips slightly parted.

Repeat three times without stopping.

Double Angle Pose

(Dwi Konasana)
(**Dwi**, two; **kona**, angles)

Benefits
Strengthens the upper spine and shoulder blades, and develops the chest and neck.

Basic position
Stand straight with your feet together, arms extended behind your back, and fingers interlocked.

Instructions
Bend forward from the waist, and stretch your arms upward and forward as far as possible.
Try to keep your neck muscles relaxed and your forehead pointing toward your knees.
Your legs should be straight as you hold the stretch.
Hold for a slow count of ten.
Slowly return to an upright position.
Repeat five times.

Breathing
Inhale before you start.
Exhale while bending.
Breathe normally while stretching.
Inhale as you return to your starting position.

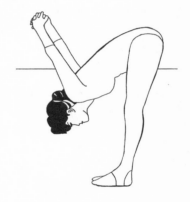

CHART YOUR PROGRESS - Degree of difficulty																	
	Hard					Easy				Hard						Easy	
Date	1	2	3	4	5	6	7	8	Date	1	2	3	4	5	6	7	8

Chart Your Progress
Body Awareness

Double Angle Pose

Date

_____

_____

_____

_____

_____

_____

_____

_____

_____

_____

_____

_____

_____

_____

_____

_____

_____

_____

_____

The Fish
(Matsyasana)

Benefits
Strengthens the abdominal muscles,
helps recirculate stagnant blood, and aids
in regulating the thyroid gland.

Basic position
Lie flat on the floor with your arms at
your sides.

Instructions
Arch your back.
Slide your hands under your buttocks.
Tilt your head back until the top of your
head rests on the floor.
Remain in the posture as long as you
comfortably can.
Slowly return to the basic position.
Repeat four or five times.

Breathing
Breathe deeply and slowly in the posture.

Variation
The instructions are the same as for the
original posture, except that the legs are
bent at the knees and the lower legs are
crossed.

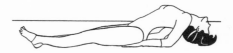

Basic posture

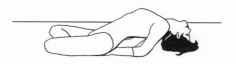

Variation

CHART YOUR PROGRESS - Degree of difficulty

Date	Hard							Easy	Date	Hard							Easy
	1	2	3	4	5	6	7	8		1	2	3	4	5	6	7	8

Chart Your Progress
Body Awareness

The Fish

Date

Your Program

Warm-ups
Sun salutation
Head rolls
Shoulder rotations
Foot exercises
Shoulder clasp
Spinal rock
The Butterfly

Breathing exercises
Complete breath
Choose additional breathing
  exercises as desired.

Asanas
Double angle pose
The Fish

Shavasana

Additional Notes

Insight

Coordinating Your Mind and Body in Harmony

When you move into and out of a posture, do it with your mind as well as with your body. Concentrate on your position, on the stretch, and on the feeling the stretch produces. If you have complete concentration throughout your exercises you will benefit from them far more than if you do them casually. By moving slowly and rhythmically, your mind will have a better chance to concentrate on the stretch and on the stillness of your body during the asana.

It is important to remember that you do not have to strain or struggle to achieve a more extreme position. You will experience greater satisfaction with your progress when you are relaxed mentally and physically, making all of your movements as easy as possible.

To experience the full benefit of the postures, allow a short rest in **savasana** after the conclusion of practice. As you rest, your mind and body will absorb the results of the stretch.

Chapter 4

New Understandings:
Regaining Your Vitality Through Relaxation

Asanas
Foot-Balancing Pose (**Padaviramasana**)
Upright Head-to-Knee Pose (**Utthita Janu Sirshasana**)

Insight:
The Benefits of Relaxing with Music

New Understandings
Regain Your Vitality Through Relaxation

Learning to attain a state of deep relaxation is one of the most important benefits to be derived from a study of yoga. Deep relaxation contributes to a sense of well-being and high energy by counteracting the stresses and tensions in your life. The word relaxation comes from the Latin **laxare**, which means "to loosen, slacken, or soften." As you already know, stress is not something that comes from the outside. It is a condition that you produce internally, of which you might not be completely aware. For example, when you lie down to rest or to sleep, your muscles may continue to carry a certain amount of residual tension. Often this tension is unnoticed, but it still can be a constant drain on your energy reserves.

A useful corollary to this is that if you create tension, you can also learn to control it with relaxation training. Therefore, although it may be difficult to control the amount of stress you experience each day, it is possible to control your response to that stress. Once you start to observe and let go of your tensions voluntarily, the process of relaxation will become more and more automatic, which, in turn, will allow you to begin to use your body in a more efficient way.

A scientific definition of deep relaxation involves the complete absence of neuromuscular activity, and includes the most beneficial kind of rest and replenishment for your mind and body. This type of relaxation can be developed by repeatedly performing the following exercises (all of the exercises, except exercise 4, should be done in **savasana**, the corpse pose as pictured in Chapter 2).

Exercise 1.

Tense all of the muscles in your feet and legs. Hold the tension briefly, and then let it go.

Slowly move your feet and legs as necessary to release the excess tension.

Let your hips sink down to a relaxed position.

Concentrate on your stomach and back. Tense the muscles and then relax them.

Pull your shoulders up by your ears. Feel the tension in your shoulders and upper back and then let it slowly drain away. Tense all of the muscles in your arms, hands, and fingers. When you have examined the tension let it fade away.

Tense the muscles in your neck and face. Feel all of the muscles that wrinkle and frown.

Let the tension go and feel the smoothness of these muscles. Concentrate on your breathing and you will become relaxed and comfortable.

When you wish to become active again, take a deep breath, stretch, and slowly come to a sitting position.

Exercise 2.

Spend a few minutes relaxing your muscles and focusing on your breathing. When you are ready, visualize any tension or illness that you are carrying. Your visualization can be anything that you would like it to be; for example, a dark stain or a color. Visualize a white light just above your head. Allow it to enter your body and slowly work its way all through you, erasing the tension or illness. When you are ready to become active again, let the light fade, taking the tension with it. Take several deep breaths, stretch, and slowly come to a sitting position.

Exercise 3.

Consciously relax your feet and lower legs, then your thighs. Let your hips sink comfortably down, and carry the relaxation to your stomach and back muscles. Take several deep breaths and continue breathing deeply throughout your relaxation. Relax your chest, your shoulders, and all of the muscles in your arms, hands, wrists, and fingers. Relax your neck, throat, and facial muscles. Feel complete relaxation in your scalp and forehead. At first this exercise is sufficient to practice alone. As you gain the ability to remove muscle tension you might try to add one of the following visualizations (choose just one each time you do this exercise). You are not limited to these; as you continue to deepen your relaxation response with practice, you will find that your imagination will provide you with many different images. After each relaxation be sure to breathe slowly and deeply several times and to stretch fully before sitting up.

Visualize a cloud drifting in the sky. Hold this image for some time and then imagine that you are the cloud. Feel light and relaxed as you float in the sky. You glide over a pleasant and familiar countryside. Feel free and airy in the vast blue sky. Stay in the visualization for as long as you wish.

Visualize a beautiful place that you know and love. Picture all of the things that you will find there. For example, if you are walking on a beach, imagine the feel of the sand. Feel the sun on your skin. See the water and the sky, and other people who might also be there. Enjoy your ability to walk in such a perfect place. Stay in the visualization for long as you wish.

Visualize an electrical current circulating around your body. It moves up your back from your heels, over your head, and down the front of your body to your toes. With practice, the current might change colors to include all of the colors of the rainbow. Continue the relaxation for as long as you wish.

Foot-Balancing Pose
(Padaviramasana)
(Pada, foot; virama, balancing)

Benefits
Strengthens the back, stomach, legs, and feet, and helps to develop balance and correct posture.

Basic position
Stand with your feet approximately four to six inches apart.
Distribute the weight of your body evenly
on both feet, arms comfortably at your sides.

Instructions
Gently lift your arms ahead of you; your elbows may be slightly bent for balance.
Simultaneously, rise up onto your toes.
Hold the asana as long as you comfortably can.
Slowly return to your original position.
Repeat between five and ten times.

Breathing
Inhale as you raise your heels and stretch out your arms.
Breathe normally in the asana.
Exhale as you lower your heels and your arms.

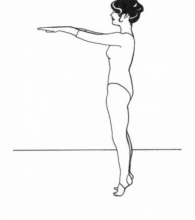

CHART YOUR PROGRESS - Degree of difficulty

Date	Hard 1	2	3	4	5	6	7	Easy 8	Date	Hard 1	2	3	4	5	6	7	Easy 8

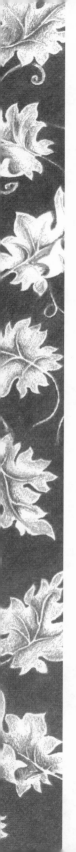

Chart Your Progress
Body Awareness

Foot-Balancing Pose

Date
_____

_____

_____

_____

_____

_____

_____

_____

_____

_____

_____

_____

_____

_____

_____

_____

_____

_____

Upright Head-to-Knee Pose

(Utthita Janu Sirshasana)
(Utthita, upright; janu: knee; sirsa, head)

Benefits

Stimulates the pancreas, relaxes the hamstring muscles and hip joints, massages the spinal nerves and brings a rich blood supply to the brain.

Basic position

Stand straight with your feet comfortably apart.
Extend your arms straight in front of you.

Instructions

Bend forward and place your hands next to your feet, or clasp your hands behind your legs.
Bring your head as close as possible into the space between your knees.
Your legs should remain as straight as possible throughout the stretch.
Hold between five and ten seconds.
Slowly return to your original position.
Repeat five times.

Breathing

Inhale deeply and exhale fully before bending.
Exhale while bending.
Breathe normally in the complete stretch.
Inhale as you straighten up.

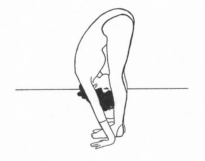

CHART YOUR PROGRESS - Degree of difficulty																	
	Hard						Easy			Hard							Easy
Date	1	2	3	4	5	6	7	8	Date	1	2	3	4	5	6	7	8

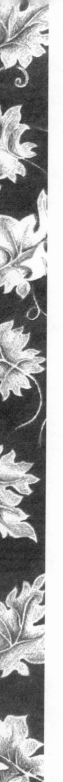

Chart Your Progress
Body Awareness

Upright Head-to-Knee Pose

Date

Your Program

Warm-ups
Sun salutation
Head rolls
Shoulder rotations
Foot exercises
Shoulder clasp
Spinal rock
The Butterfly

Breathing exercises
Complete breath
Choose additional breathing
  exercises as desired.

Asanas
Double angle pose
The Fish
Foot-balancing pose
Upright head-to-knee pose

Shavasana

Additional Notes

_____

_____

_____

_____

_____

_____

_____

_____

_____

_____

_____

_____

_____

_____

_____

_____

_____

Insight

The Benefits of Relaxing With Music

Using music to create a deep state of relaxation is extremely beneficial. Music allows you to move into another dimension where you are more aware of the sounds you hear than you are of the stresses and tensions that you habitually carry. The act of listening to soothing music allows your muscles to relax and your mind to become peaceful and calm. Since each person responds differently to music, it is important to select pieces that are peaceful and soothing to you. When you listen to music for the purpose of relaxation, you should set aside fifteen minutes or more of uninterrupted time.

Once you have selected the music, allow your body to relax in a comfortable position with your eyes closed. If you focus your attention on the music, you will find that your cares and worries begin to drift away. Mentally scan your body, noticing when areas of tension begin to diminish and release as you become more deeply relaxed. When the music ends, scan your body again, and become aware of how relaxed you feel. With regular practice, your relaxation will become easier and deeper.

If you would like to start a record or tape library of music for relaxation, you will find New Age music available from metaphysical book and music stores around the country. Look for them in your telephone directory.

Chapter 5

New Understandings:
Yin, Yang, and the Flow of Prana

Asanas
Leg Pulls (**Supta Padasana**)
Shoulder Stand (**Sarvangasana**)

Insight:
How You Become Your Thoughts

New Understandings
Yin, Yang, and the Flow of Prana

Just as the seasons change and the night follows the day, yoga teaches that within all forms of nature are two opposing energy forces constantly interacting and interchanging. The first represents negativity—cold, darkness, shade, and passiveness; the second represents positiveness—heat, light, sunshine, and activity. Within this belief system, which is still widely held in China, Japan, and India, the contraction and expansion of these forces is thought to be the source of the energy that animates all living things. Of utmost importance in yogic philosophy is the establishment of a balance and harmony between negative and positive energy, not only in a cosmic sense but in the sense of personal inner harmony, centeredness, and growth.

This vital energy is called **chi** by the Chinese, **ki** by the Japanese, and **prana** in India. Within the yogic tradition, individual pranic energy or life force and universal energy are seen to be the same as you surround a small portion of the energy of the universe with your body and say, "This is me."

In yogic philosophy it is seen that since nature always tends toward balance, eventually everything becomes its opposite. This theory is illustrated by the symbol of yin (negative energy) and yang (positive energy). The dynamic curve dividing them suggests that they are continuously merging. Thus, yin and yang create each other, transform into each other, and depend on each other for definition.

YIN	YANG
Negative	Positive
Passive	Active
Female	Male
Receptive	Creative
Dark	Light
Night	Day
Cold	Heat
Soft	Hard
Wet	Dry
Winter	Summer
Shadow	Sun

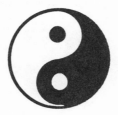

Yoga teaches that it is of utmost importance for us to recognize the ways in which we may be blocking the source of our energy and healing. By failing to understand fully the natural pattern of life and thereby blocking it, we may be causing unnecessary problems and illnesses. Conversely, by becoming open to the flow of prana, to the flow of life, we can bring happiness and a deep sense of peace to ourselves and to those around us.

Leg Pulls

(Supta Padasana)
(**Supta**, supine; **pada**, foot)

Benefits
Firms the abdomen, buttocks, and thighs, limbers leg muscles, and stretches the spine.

Basic position
Lie on your back, arms relaxed at your sides.

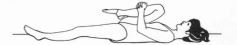

Position 1

Instructions
Bend your right leg and pull it close to your body.
Be sure that your left leg is extended in a straight line from your hips to your toes.
Raise your right leg.
When it is fully extended, pull your foot back as far as you can without straining.
Slowly return to your original position.
Repeat five times with each leg.

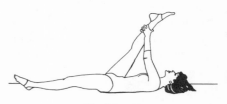

Breathing
Breathe normally as you do this asana.

Position 2

CHART YOUR PROGRESS - Degree of difficulty

	Hard							Easy		Hard							Easy
Date	1	2	3	4	5	6	7	8	Date	1	2	3	4	5	6	7	8

Chart Your Progress
Body Awareness
Leg Pulls

Date

Shoulder Stand

(Sarvangasana)
(Sarva, whole; anga, body)

Benefits
Stimulates the thyroid gland, improves the balance of the circulatory and digestive systems, brings blood to the brain, and tones the legs, abdomen, spine, and neck.

Basic position
Lie flat on your back with your feet together, arms at your sides, and palms flat on the floor.

Instructions
Place your hands behind your back for balance.
Bring your knees close to your ears.
When you have your balance, slowly extend your legs and back to a vertical position.
Continue steadying your body with the palms of your hands.
Your body and legs should extend straight upward, forming a right angle with your neck and shoulders.
Your chest and chin should be close together.
Hold the asana as long as you comfortably can.
Slowly return to the basic position.
Repeat five times.

Breathing
Inhale.
Retain the breath inside while assuming and returning from this posture.
Breathe normally while in the raised position.

Limitations
Do not do this asana if you have high blood pressure or a heart condition.

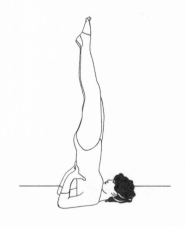

CHART YOUR PROGRESS - Degree of difficulty																
	Hard						Easy			Hard						Easy
Date	1	2	3	4	5	6	7	8	Date	1	2	3	4	5	6	7	8

Variation

The instructions are the same as in the original position except that the chin is not pressed against the chest in the final pose, and the trunk is held at a forty-five-degree angle to the floor instead of at a right angle. This posture is easier and is recommended for beginners.

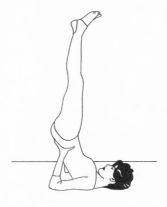

CHART YOUR PROGRESS - Degree of difficulty

	Hard						Easy			Hard						Easy
Date	1	2	3	4	5	6	7	8	Date	1	2	3	4	5	6	7	8

Chart Your Progress
Body Awareness

Shoulder Stand

Date

Your Program

Warm-ups
Sun salutation
Head rolls
Shoulder rotations
Foot exercises
Shoulder clasp
Spinal rock
The Butterfly

Breathing exercises
Complete breath
Choose additional breathing
  exercises as desired.

Asanas
Double angle pose
The Fish
Foot-balancing pose
Upright head-to-knee pose
Leg pulls
Shoulder stand

Shavasana

Additional Notes

_____

_____

_____

_____

_____

_____

_____

_____

_____

_____

_____

_____

_____

_____

_____

_____

_____

Insight

How You Become Your Thoughts

Just as the food you eat eventually reaches your bloodstream and nourishes all of the cells of your body, your thoughts are the food that nourishes your mind. Thoughts can determine the whole character of your life, and it is the subjects that you allow your mind to dwell on that make you and your surroundings what they are.

Yogic philosophy includes the realization that thought is the real causative force in life. The belief that you choose all the conditions of your life when you choose your thoughts has been the subject of many yogic scholarly studies.

The yogi believes that if you change your thoughts your conditions must also change. Positive thoughts bring about corresponding positive conditions, whereras negative thoughts bring about corresponding negative conditions. Therefore, it is important to assess your habitual thoughts to discover whether they are contributing to your happiness or detracting from the quality of your life.

One of the best ways to understand the many ways your thoughts affect the outcomes of each and every day is to begin to pay special attention to your "mental tapes." You can, if you wish, gain greater insight into your thought patterns by using the following pages to write down things that come into your mind consistently and repetitively.

Mental Tapes

Mental Tapes

Chapter 6

New Understandings:
The Blessedness of Good Sleep

Asanas
The Boat (**Naukasana**)
Shoulder Pose or Bridge (**Kandharasana**)

Insight:
Seven Days to New Ways of Thinking

New Understandings
The Blessedness of Good Sleep

When your sleep is deep and restful you wake up in the morning feeling refreshed and ready to begin a new day. You will find that the stretching, breathing, and relaxation exercises of yoga will greatly enhance your ability to enjoy the results of a sound sleep every night.

If you have difficulty falling asleep, several helpful yogic practices will aid you to drift into a pleasant sleep easily and comfortably. These same techniques also apply whenever you awaken during the night and wish to go back to sleep.

Three yogic rules encourage good sleep habits. First, make sure that your sleeping surface is firm and that your head is only slightly raised to permit good circulation. Second, try not to eat for at least two hours before retiring, because you will sleep better if your digestive system is not active. If you want something before bedtime, a piece of fruit or a glass of warm milk would be the best choice. Finally, sleep in a room that is well ventilated and cool, with adequate bed covering to make you comfortable. Clothing should not bind or restrict you in any way.

When you are certain that all of your physical requirements have been met, it is time to quiet your mind and body. Just as you set a physical climate favorable for sleep, try to develop a mental climate that is conducive to deep rest and relaxation. You will find that you can fall asleep easily and comfortably when you have learned the methods that work for you. The following suggestions might help.

Create a sleep tape from the relaxation exercises in Chapter 4. That chapter also suggests that soothing music can help you achieve a deep state of physical and mental relaxation. Choose a mantra (Chapter 11) to repeat as you drift into sleep. When the mantra is combined with deep breathing, sleep soon comes easily.

Learn to direct your focus and become "one-pointed." With your eyes closed, focus on one spot with complete concentration. This technique will limit the distractions that hinder your ability to sleep. Just before retiring it might be helpful to do a few asanas such as the back stretch, the cobra, and the plow. Also, you may wish to include any of the breathing exercises found in Chapter 3.

The Boat

(Naukasana)
(Nauk, boat)

Benefits
Strengthens the legs, stomach, and back
muscles, and tones the abdominal
organs.

Basic position
Sit on the floor with your back straight,
your knees bent, and your feet together.

Instructions
Extend your arms forward in line with
your shoulders.
Slowly straighten and lift your legs until
you are balancing on your buttocks.
Hold your balance as long as you com-
fortably can.
Gently return to the basic position.
Repeat two to four times.

Breathing
Inhale as you begin the asana.
Retain the breath while balancing.
Exhale as you release the posture.

Limitation
Do not attempt the boat pose if you have
a lower back problem.

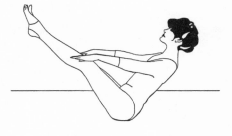

CHART YOUR PROGRESS - Degree of difficulty																	
	Hard							Easy		Hard							Easy
Date	1	2	3	4	5	6	7	8	Date	1	2	3	4	5	6	7	8

Chart Your Progress
Body Awareness

The Boat

Date

Bridge or Shoulder Pose

(Kandharasana)
(Kandhar, shoulder)

Benefits

Strengthens the arms, wrists, and lower back, limbers the spine, and stretches the female organs and assists in preventing menstrual cramps.

Basic position

Lie flat on your back with your knees bent and your feet about a shoulder-width apart. Keep your arms relaxed at your sides.

Instructions

Slowly raise your buttocks and arch your back.

Keep your heels on the floor, and place your hands firmly under your back for support.

Your body should be supported by your feet, head, neck, shoulders, and upper arms.

Hold the posture as long as you comfortably can.

Slowly return to the basic position.

Repeat three to five times.

After your last stretch (to avoid back problems) lie on your back and hug your knees for a full minute or more.

Breathing

Inhale as you establish the position. Breathe deeply while holding the posture. Exhale as you return to your starting position.

Limitation

Do not do this asana during menstruation.

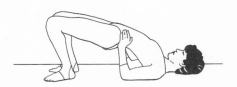

CHART YOUR PROGRESS - Degree of difficulty																	
	Hard							Easy		Hard							Easy
Date	1	2	3	4	5	6	7	8	Date	1	2	3	4	5	6	7	8

VARIATIONS

Variation 1

The instructions are the same as for the
original posture except that the right
knee is bent toward the chest and the leg
is fully extended. You may wish to flex
and point your foot while in the stretch.

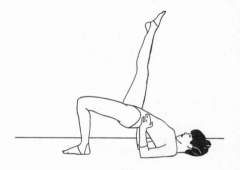

Variation 1

CHART YOUR PROGRESS - Degree of difficulty

	Hard							Easy		Hard							Easy
Date	1	2	3	4	5	6	7	8	Date	1	2	3	4	5	6	7	8

Variation 2

The instructions are the same for the original posture except that the arms are flat on the floor and the hands are around the ankles. The feet should be held at least a shoulder-width apart.

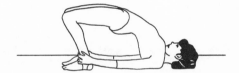

Variation 2

CHART YOUR PROGRESS - Degree of difficulty

Date	Hard 1	2	3	4	5	6	7	Easy 8	Date	Hard 1	2	3	4	5	6	7	Easy 8

Chart Your Progress
Body Awareness

Bridge or Shoulder Pose

Date

Your Program

Warm-ups
Sun salutation
Head rolls
Shoulder rotations
Foot exercises
Shoulder clasp
Spinal rock
The Butterfly

Breathing exercises
Complete breath
Choose additional breathing
 exercises as desired.

Asanas
Double angle pose
The Fish
Foot-balancing pose
Upright head-to-knee pose
Leg pulls
Shoulder stand
The Boat
The Bridge

Shavasana

Additional Notes

Insight

Seven Days to New Ways of Thinking

Now that you have a better idea of your usual thoughts, it is time to discover a very effective way to acquire new thought patterns to replace the negative ones. By following the seven-day mental diet you will be amazed at the interesting things that you will learn about yourself. You can expect to get results almost from the beginning.

Make up your mind to devote one week solely to the task of building a new habit of thought, and let everything else in your life become unimportant in comparison. This does not simply mean that you will be able to face your present difficulties in a better spirit; it means that the difficulties will change for the better.

For seven days you must not allow yourself to dwell for a single moment on any kind of negative thought. Watch carefully and do not, under any pretense, allow your mind to dwell on anything that is not positive, constructive, optimistic, and kind. This discipline will be so strenuous that you could not maintain it consciously for much more than a week. At the end of that time your habit of positive thinking will begin to be established. Some extraordinary changes for the better will have come into your life. The new way of thinking will be so attractive and so much easier than the old way that you will not wish to change back.

Do not begin the seven-day mental diet lightly. Think about it for a while before you begin. If you make a false start, stop for several days and then begin again. Giving up food is much easier than giving up thoughts you have become accustomed to, even though they are negative.

When you begin the diet, all kinds of thoughts will seem to be stirred up and negatives will fly at you from all directions, but that is an encouraging sign. It means that your world is moving and changing. If you are able to hang on, the moving and changing will pass, leaving your life reassembled into something much closer to your real desire.

During this week you will possibly want something to aid you. It will be of help to picture yourself securely held by a large stable rock. Your world may shake violently but the rock will remain secure. Every time a negative thought enters your mind, think of it as a cigarette ash and flick it off immediately. If an ash stays even a second it burns. Every possible negative will try to enter your mind; remember that it may enter, but you will not let it remain. The thoughts that you dwell on are the ones that can harm or help you.

Think of your experience as a challenge, because that is what it will certainly be. Having been challenged you will experience a great feeling of accomplishment when you are finished. It takes someone who wants to change his or her life from negative to positive, someone very determined, to complete the entire week of the diet.

Chapter 7

New Understandings:
Yoga, Sports, and You

Asanas
The Lion (**Simhasana**)
The Triangle (**Trikonasana**)

Insight:
The Magic of Palming

New Understandings
Yoga, Sports, and You

The consistent practice of yoga brings about a state of increased flexibility and strength where natural movement can occur spontaneously. Once you have rediscovered flexibility and proper body alignment, you will find that most of your movements have become smoother and take less energy to perform.

The yogic ideal of movement encourages the body to move with its own natural momentum and grace. The human body, like that of any animal, has an intelligence of its own and will move easily and spontaneously when it is allowed to do so.

We have all encountered someone who is a natural athlete, who displays a sense of agility, looseness, relaxation, and nimbleness. These are all qualities that cannot be taught. They come from within when the body's inner resources have not been suppressed.

Through yoga you can acquire the skills that allow your mind and body to function together in harmony. For example, while competing in a sport you may experience anxiety or tension when confronted with a strong desire to win. When you regularly practice the yogic relaxation and mental centering exercises, however, you will discover that the act of winning does not require your specific concentration. Your awareness will be on the play as it is happening. By developing an attitude that allows you to concentrate on each moment as it occurs, rather than on a past error or fear of a future one, you will have a greater chance of achieving the win and have the additional satisfaction of enjoying your participation. Whether you plan to compete in a sport or simply enrich your life with new skills for your leisure time, the yogic body movement and mental centering practices will help you to attain your goals in a new and rewarding way.

The Lion
(Simhasana)
(Simha, lion)

Benefits
Firms the muscles of the face and neck,
sends extra blood to the throat, and massages and tones the neck muscles and
ligaments.

Basic position
Sit cross-legged or in the half-lotus position.

Instructions
Place your hands over your knees with
the fingers spread apart.
Extend your tongue outward and down-
ward as far as you can.
At the same time, open your eyes wide.
Hold for as long as comfortable.
Slowly return to the beginning position.
Repeat four times.

Breathing
Inhale before starting the posture.
Exhale slowly while in the posture.
You may also produce a clear and steady
"ah" sound as you exhale.

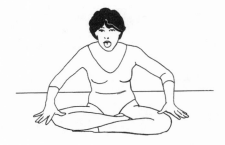

CHART YOUR PROGRESS - Degree of difficulty

Date	Hard 1	2	3	4	5	6	7	Easy 8	Date	Hard 1	2	3	4	5	6	7	Easy 8

Chart Your Progress
Body Awareness

The Lion

Date
_____

_____

_____

_____

_____

_____

_____

_____

_____

_____

_____

_____

_____

_____

_____

The Triangle Pose
(Trikonasana)
(Trikon, triangle)

Benefits
Stimulates the nervous system, improves
digestion, gently massages the spinal
nerves and muscles of the lower back,
and abdominal organs.

Basic position
Stand with your legs wide apart.
Turn your left foot out approximately
ninety degrees and your right foot in
approximately thirty degrees.
Be sure that the heel of your left foot is
directly in line with the middle of your
right foot.
Raise your arms to shoulder level.

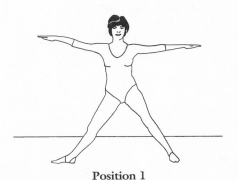

Position 1

Instructions
Bend from the hip slowly to the left side,
keeping both of your hips in an even line.
Bring your left hand to your ankle or
calf, or where you can reach, without
straining.
Extend your right arm vertically and, if
you wish, look up at your hand.
Do not be discouraged if at first you do
not reach the completed stretch.
Slowly return to the basic position.
Repeat on the other side. (Be sure to
change the foot position.)
Repeat three times on each side.

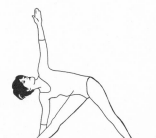

Position 2

Breathing
Inhale while raising your arms.
Exhale while bending to the side.
Hold your breath out while stretching.

CHART YOUR PROGRESS - Degree of difficulty																	
	Hard						Easy			Hard							Easy
Date	1	2	3	4	5	6	7	8	Date	1	2	3	4	5	6	7	8

Chart Your Progress
Body Awareness

The Triangle

Date

_____

_____

_____

_____

_____

_____

_____

_____

_____

_____

_____

_____

_____

_____

_____

_____

_____

Your Program

Warm-ups
Sun salutation
Head rolls
Shoulder rotations
Foot exercises
Shoulder clasp
Spinal rock
The Butterfly

Breathing exercises
Complete breath
Choose additional
 breathing exercises as desired.

Asanas
Double angle pose
The Fish
Foot-balancing pose
Upright head-to-knee
 pose
Leg pulls
Shoulder stand
The Boat
The Bridge
The Lion
The Triangle

Shavasana

Additional Notes

Insight

The Magic of Palming

This exercise, referred to as palming or cupping, not only has a most relaxing effect on your eyes and your entire nervous system, but also greatly improves vision blurred by tension or fatigue. Instead of reaching for that extra cup of coffee when you are tired, try this exercise.

Sit upright. If you wish, place your elbows on a table, using a book or pillow to allow you to keep your elbows on the table without lowering your head.

Briskly rub your palms together until you feel warmth. Cup your hands over your eyes so that your palms directly cover your closed eyelids. Keep your fingers crossed on your forehead.

In this position do deep rhythmic breathing for a short while, then resume your normal breathing. Continue for several more minutes. It is important to be relaxed and comfortable, but with your spine straight and your head upright. When your neck is bent the free flow of blood is impeded and the flow of life energy is impaired or constricted.

Palming is a very relaxing and soothing exercise that you can practice any time and place.

Chapter 8

New Understandings:
How to Use Yoga Throughout Your Day

Asanas
The Locust (**Shalabhasana**)
The Bow (**Dhanurasana**)

Insight:
The Peaceful Prayer Pose Meditation

New Understandings
How to Use Yoga Throughout Your Day

Several commercial airlines recently published their recommendations on how you can avoid the exhausting effects of lengthy flights. They suggest that you do deep breathing exercises, stretch as often as possible, and move the major muscles in a slow, rhythmic way. In other words, you should use the concepts of yoga. Although this art is more than six thousand years old, it is as modern as today in application. We don't have to look far to see how practicing it will be of benefit to you all day long. As you progress throughout your day, try to keep the following points in mind.

Whenever you feel like it, stretch. Stretching is tranquilizing. You can avoid those kinks and cramps if you stretch before tension and tightness take over.

Breathe deeply all day.

Caught in rush-hour traffic, you can reduce stress by breathing deeply, repeating your mantra and doing head, shoulder, and neck rotations.

At any convenient time you can flex and contract your muscles, the better to relax afterward.

The Locust Pose
(Shalabhasana)
(Shalabha, locust)

Benefits
Beneficial for all the abdominal organs,
acts on the intestines aiding digestion
and elimination, and strengthens the
lower back.

Basic position
Lie on your stomach with your hands in
a
fist under your thighs to give leverage.
Your chin should be touching the floor.

Instructions
Stretch your legs and tense your arms.
Raise your legs as high as possible with-
out bending them.
Hold the position for as long as you
wish.
Slowly return to your original position.
Repeat three to five times.

Breathing
Inhale before you start.
Hold your breath while raising your legs.
Exhale while returning to the starting
position.

Limitations
Do not practice the locust if you have an
ulcer, hernia, or lower back problems.

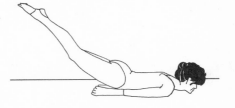

CHART YOUR PROGRESS - Degree of difficulty

Date	Hard 1	2	3	4	5	6	7	Easy 8	Date	Hard 1	2	3	4	5	6	7	Easy 8

Variation

The instructions are the same as for the original posture except that one leg is raised and the other is kept fully extended on the floor.

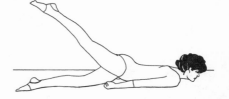

CHART YOUR PROGRESS - Degree of difficulty																	
	Hard							Easy		Hard							Easy
Date	1	2	3	4	5	6	7	8	Date	1	2	3	4	5	6	7	8

Chart Your Progress
Body Awareness

The Locust

Date

_____

_____

_____

_____

_____

_____

_____

_____

_____

_____

_____

_____

_____

_____

_____

_____

_____

_____

The Bow

(Dhanurasana)
(Dhanu, bow)

Benefits
Massages the abdominal organs and muscles, and aids digestion and elimination.

Basic position
Lie flat on your stomach with your arms at your sides.

Instructions
Bend your knees and hold onto your ankles.
Arch your back.
Using the strength of your arm muscles, pull back on your ankles as you raise your head, chest, and thighs.
Look up as high as you can.
Be sure to keep your arms straight.
Hold the position as long as you comfortably can.
Slowly and carefully return to the basic position.
Repeat between three and five times.
After you last stretch, to avoid back problems, lie on your back and hug your knees for a full minute or more.

Breathing
Inhale as you stretch into the posture.
Breathe deeply during the stretch.
Exhale as you slowly return to the basic position.

Limitations
Do not practice the bow if you have ulcers, hernia, or lower back pain.

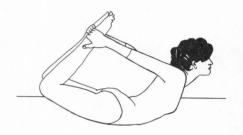

CHART YOUR PROGRESS - Degree of difficulty

Date	Hard 1	2	3	4	5	6	7	Easy 8	Date	Hard 1	2	3	4	5	6	7	Easy 8

Variation

The instructions are the same as for the original posture except that you do not arch your back or raise your legs as high. This is the recommended posture for beginners.

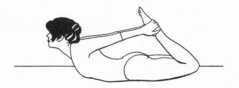

CHART YOUR PROGRESS - Degree of difficulty

Date	Hard 1	2	3	4	5	6	7	Easy 8	Date	Hard 1	2	3	4	5	6	7	Easy 8

Chart Your Progress
Body Awareness

The Bow

Date

Your Program

Warm-ups
Sun salutation
Head rolls
Shoulder rotations
Foot exercises
Shoulder clasp
Spinal rock
The Butterfly

Breathing exercises
Complete breath
Choose additional breathing
  exercises as desired.

Asanas
Double angle pose
The Fish
Foot-balancing pose
Upright head-to-knee pose
Leg pulls
Shoulder stand
The Boat
The Bridge
The Lion
The Triangle
The Locust
The Bow

Shavasana

Additional Notes

Insight

The Peaceful Prayer Pose Meditation

One of the principal benefits that can be derived from a study of yoga is learning simple techniques that will allow you to feel centered and grounded within a short period of time. The prayer pose meditation will not only help you to ease the tensions in your daily life, but will also provide a useful tool for becoming peaceful, centered, comfortably relaxed, and in harmony with your inner self.

This meditation is based on the fact that a slight pressure on the sternum, between the breasts at the level of the heart, produces a feeling of ease and calmness. It is the acupuncture point called the "sea of tranquility" and is thought by acupuncturists to be the most centering point in the body.

Sit with your back straight and your head upright. Place your palms together and press slightly against your chest between your breasts. Close your eyes and take slow deep breaths. Send your breath into your chest and experience a warmth and calmness within your heart.

Chapter 9

New Understandings:
The Ancient Sanskrit Language

Asanas:
Cat Stretch (**Marjariasana**)
Head-to-Knee Pose (**Janushirasana**)

Insight:
Looking at Your New Dimensions

New Understandings
The Ancient Sanskrit Language

Most of the terminology used in yoga is from Sanskrit. As you learn the asanas and study the philosophy of yoga, you will encounter many Sanskrit words and their translations.

Sanskrit is one of humanity's oldest languages. It belongs to the Indo-European group of languages that also includes English, Welsh, Latin, and Greek. The original Indo-European speakers were tribes inhabiting the plains of Eastern Europe in the third millennium B.C. Specifically, the evolution of this language belongs to the Indo-Iranian tribes known as Aryans from the name they gave themselves (Sanskrit-arya) and from which the modern name Iran is derived. The name Eire for Ireland is also thought to have the same origin.

The main movement of Aryan migration was into Central Asia, and from there by separate migrations into Iran and India. Thereafter, the Aryans of Iran and the Aryans of India went their separate ways both culturally and linguistically. The speech introduced by the Aryans into India developed into what we now call Sanskrit.

The first written account of Sanskrit is attributed to the Indian Paniei, who wrote a grammar recording and standardizing the language in the fourth century B.C. By that time, Sanskrit had become the language of the educated classes, although many regional dialects were still in use. Sanskrit was the language of scholarly works and of scientific inquiry, including learned discussions in medical schools. It is in this language that we find most of the texts from ancient and medieval India.

The word Sanskrit (**samskrta**) means "polished, grammatically correct." Because of the long recorded history of the language and the many sources from which it drew its vocabulary, it is rich in its variety of descriptive words. Every expression has many different meanings. The Sanskrit word for karma, for example, means "individuality," "character," "act," "deed," and also "destiny."

With the advent of modern education, Sanskrit slowly tended to become a specialized subject of study, rather than a normal element of the culture of the educated classes. Compositions in the language, however, continue to be produced in every literary form. Since it continues to be written, although in decreasing volume, its literary tradition may be said to extend for three thousand years.

Cat Stretch

(**Marjariasana**)
(**Marjari**, cat)

Benefits
Stretches and massages the back, tones the muscles of the back, neck, shoulders, abdomen, and spine, and aids in spinal flexibility.

Basic position
Rest your weight on your hands and knees.

Instructions
Slowly depress your spine and raise your head.
Lower your head and arch your back.
Continue raising and lowering your back and head slowly for five repetitions.

Breathing
Inhale before you start.
Exhale as you arch your spine.
Inhale as you depress your spine.

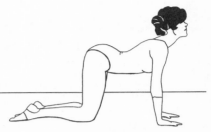

Position 1

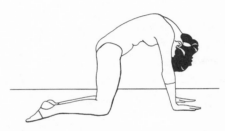

Position 2

CHART YOUR PROGRESS - Degree of difficulty																
	Hard						Easy			Hard						Easy
Date	1	2	3	4	5	6	7	8	Date	1	2	3	4	5	6	7	8

Chart Your Progress
Body Awareness

Cat Stretch

Date

Head-to-Knee Pose

(Janushirasana)
(Janu, knee; sirsa, head)

Benefits
Stretches the hamstring muscles, tones the abdomen, and encourages a fresh supply of blood to the spinal nerves and muscles.

Basic position
Sit on the floor with your legs straight. Rest your hands on your thighs.

Instructions
Fold one leg and place your heel against your thigh.
Lean forward and gently hold the toes of your straight leg with both hands.
If you cannot reach your toes, hold your ankle or lower leg.
Keep your leg as straight as possible without bending your knee.
Using your arms, slowly stretch your body forward so that your head is close to your straight leg.
Hold the stretch for a comfortable length of time.
Slowly return to the basic position.
Repeat on the other side.
Do two or three stretches on each side.

Breathing
Exhale while bending forward.
Breathe normally while holding the posture.
Inhale while returning to the original posture.

Limitations
Do not do this asana if you have a slipped disk, sciatica, chronic arthritis, or lower back pain.

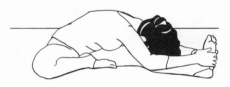

CHART YOUR PROGRESS - Degree of difficulty																	
	Hard						Easy			Hard							Easy
Date	1	2	3	4	5	6	7	8	Date	1	2	3	4	5	6	7	8

Variation

Basic position
Sit on the floor with your legs straight.
Rest your hands on your thighs.

Instructions
Extend your legs wide apart.
Slide your hands down your legs.
Hold onto your ankles, feet or toes.
Keep your legs as straight as you can.
Using your arms, slowly stretch to the
center with your back straight and flat.
Keep your head up and try to relax your
shoulders as you stretch.
Hold the stretch for a comfortable length
of time.
Slowly return to the basic position.
Do the forward stretch two or three
times.
Repeat the same stretch to the side.
Do the stretch two or three times on each
side.

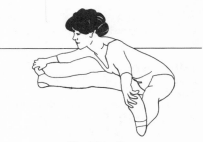

Position 1

Breathing
Exhale while bending forward.
Breathe normally while holding the pos-
ture.
Inhale while returning to the original
position.

Limitations
Do not do this asana if you have a slipped
disk, sciatica, or chronic arthritis.

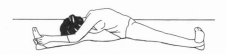

Position 2

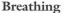

CHART YOUR PROGRESS - Degree of difficulty																	
	Hard							Easy		Hard							Easy
Date	1	2	3	4	5	6	7	8	Date	1	2	3	4	5	6	7	8

Chart Your Progress
Body Awareness

Head-to-Knee Pose

Date

Your Program

Warm-ups
Sun salutation
Head rolls
Shoulder rotations
Foot exercises
Shoulder clasp
Spinal rock
The Butterfly

Breathing exercises
Complete breath
Choose additional breathing
  exercises as desired.

Asanas
Double angle pose
The Fish
Foot-balancing pose
Upright head-to-knee pose
Leg pulls
Shoulder stand
The Boat
The Bridge
The Lion
The Triangle
The Locust
The Bow
Cat stretch
Head-to-knee pose

Shavasana

Additional Notes

_____

_____

_____

_____

_____

_____

_____

_____

_____

_____

_____

_____

_____

_____

_____

_____

_____

Insight
Look at Your New Dimensions

Congratulations! You have completed the first half of your journal and are now practicing twenty-two important exercises, many of which require the use of muscles you may not have used regularly in years, and some of which manipulate your body in ways that are totally new. At this point you can begin to judge where you are weakest (back, legs, balance, etc.) and devote a little extra attention to those areas as you continue to perform the exercises.

By now you have probably discovered that your progress in the asanas is irregular. Some days a position may seem easy to do and then the next day, or for several days, it feels difficult to achieve the same degree of stretch. The learning process in yoga can be irregular and demands that you approach each day without expectations of greater gain.

Yoga, by its very nature, is noncompetitive. When your body feels stiff and less responsive, instead of pushing or straining, the goal can only be met by letting go. What appears as a setback is really a preparation for further and greater gain when your body is ready. If you simply allow your body to move as it feels right to move and go easy without becoming discouraged when you feel stiff, your reward will be a slow but measurable gain that will last a lifetime.

Chapter 10

New Understandings:
Meditation: Awakening Your Power

Asanas
The Plow (**Halasana**)

The Cobra (**Bhujangasana**)

Insight:
Looking Further at Meditation Techniques

New Understandings
Meditation: Awakening Your Power

When you have become familiar with the basic postures and the breathing and relaxation techniques, you will be able to further understand and appreciate yoga even more by studying the concepts of meditation that are a vital part of the yogic tradition. In the West we explore the external world and create a wealth of material technology. In the East, the study of the inner world of consciousness takes precedence. Whereas Western scholars look to outer space with an inquiring mind, the yogic scholar looks to the laws of the universe with a view to expanding knowledge of inner space.

Through meditation you learn to focus uncritically on one thing at a time. This is a kind of self-discipline that increases your self-awareness and your ability to eventually discover more about your interior world. With practice, you can understand better and accept habitual patterns of perception, thought, and feeling that previously had an influence over your life without your complete awareness.

This ancient tradition has been found to be effective in creating a state of deep relaxation in a relatively short period of time. During meditation your body's metabolism is slowed, alpha brain waves are increased, and the amount of internal and external stimuli you respond to is greatly reduced.

The purpose of raja yoga meditations is to gain control over the stream of thoughts that flow through the human mind. It seeks to check the flow and still the mind by means of concentration (**dharana**) and contemplation (**dhyana**). By these practices a state of superconsciousness (**samadhi**) may be achieved. Just as a body that has been cleansed of its toxic waste becomes healthier and stronger, so a mind emptied of its encumbering thoughts becomes healthier and stronger.

The practice of meditation will be made more valuable by following these preliminary guidelines.

Prepare a clean, quiet area with adequate ventilation. Make sure that you will have at least half an hour without disturbance. Wear loose, clean clothing, and sit or lie on a clean mat or rug.

Try to meditate in the same place at the same hour each day. If you do not have twenty or thirty minutes at one time, try to meditate for fifteen minutes twice a day.

Plan your meditation with your eating needs in mind. Generally it is best to wait at least an hour after a meal. As meditation becomes a regular habit you will begin to prefer to eat lightly before or after your practice.

Regulate the flow of your breath when you begin your meditation. It is helpful initially to focus on your breath and to breathe slowly and easily. This practice also aids you in controlling the mind. As you meditate you should establish a slow, rhythmic breathing pattern that will allow your mind and body to relax into the meditation. It will soon seem as if the breathing continues on its own without your conscious awareness of a need for control.

It is traditional to rest your hands on your thighs with the tips of the thumb and index finger of each hand joined in the yogic **chin mudra** ("finger position").

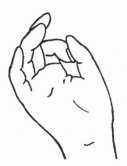

This aids your meditation by allowing the **ki** energy in the meridians to flow freely to the fingertips and back up both your arms. If you find the **chin mudra** distracting in any way, you can meditate with your hands resting comfortably in an open position on your thighs.

It is common during meditation to sit or kneel. For either position, you may use a pillow for added comfort and support. It is also possible to meditate lying down.

Maintain the posture with your back, neck, and head in a straight line, preferably facing the earth's magnetic poles to the north or east. When you meditate you should feel steady and relaxed.

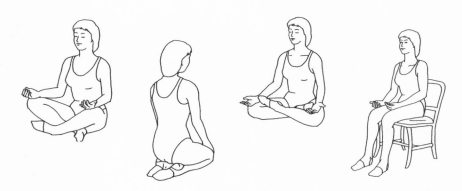

The Plow

(Halasana)
(Hala, plow)

Benefits
Stretches the spine; tones the kidneys, liver, and gallbladder; limbers the pelvis and legs; and improves digestion.

Basic position
Lie flat on your back with your arms at your sides.

Instructions
Bring your knees up to your ears and support your back with your hands. Gently extend your legs back until your toes touch the floor.
Keep your legs as straight as possible without straining and, if you wish, bring your hands gently down to the floor behind your back.
Hold the position for as long as it is comfortable.
Slowly return to the basic position using your hands to support your back.
In the beginning, if you feel unsteady in the plow, keep your hands on your back until you have gained more flexibility and confidence.
Repeat four times.

Breathing
Inhale deeply and exhale fully before starting.
Retain your breath out while rolling back.
Breathe normally in the final position.
Retain your breath out as you return to the basic position.

Limitations
Do not practice the asana if you have sciatica or lower back pain, or are menstruating heavily.

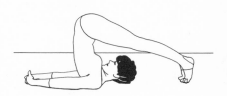

CHART YOUR PROGRESS - Degree of difficulty

	Hard						Easy			Hard						Easy
Date	1	2	3	4	5	6	7	8	Date	1	2	3	4	5	6	7	8

Chart Your Progress
Body Awareness
The Plow

Date

_____

_____

_____

_____

_____

_____

_____

_____

_____

_____

_____

_____

_____

_____

_____

_____

The Cobra
(Bhujangasana)
(Bhujanga; cobra)

Benefits
Beneficial for all the abdominal organs, especially the liver and gallbladder, keeps the spine supple and healthy, and strengthens the arm muscles.

Basic position
Lie on your stomach with your legs straight and the palms of your hands flat on the floor under your shoulders. Rest your forehead on the floor.

Instructions
Slowly raise your head and shoulders off the ground, bending your head as far back as it will go.
First, try to raise your upper body without using your arms.
Let your back muscles begin the stretch. When you have raised your body as far as you can, using your back muscles only, continue stretching back using the pressure of your arms to continue your stretch.
Stretch back until your arms are straight. Keep your hips on or close to the floor. Hold the posture as long as you comfortably can.
Slowly return to the original position. Repeat up to four times.

Breathing
Inhale while raising your body.
Breathe normally while in the final posture.
Exhale while you return to the original position.

Limitations
Do not do this asana if you have peptic ulcers or hernia.

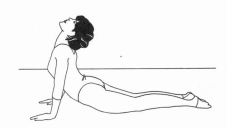

	Hard							Easy		Hard							Easy
Date	1	2	3	4	5	6	7	8	Date	1	2	3	4	5	6	7	8

Variation

Instructions are the same as for the original position except that the head is turned as far as possible to one side.
Do the variation up to four times to each side.

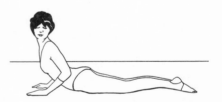

CHART YOUR PROGRESS - Degree of difficulty

Date	Hard 1	2	3	4	5	6	7	Easy 8	Date	Hard 1	2	3	4	5	6	7	Easy 8

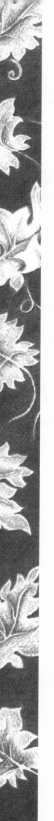

Chart Your Progress
Body Awareness

The Cobra

Date
_____

_____

_____

_____

_____

_____

_____

_____

_____

_____

_____

_____

_____

_____

_____

Your Program

Warm-ups
Sun salutation
Head rolls
Shoulder rotations
Foot exercises
Shoulder clasp
Spinal rock
The Butterfly

Breathing exercises
Complete breath
Choose additional breathing
  exercises as desired.

Asanas
Double angle pose
The Fish
Foot-balancing pose
Upright head-to-knee pose
Leg pulls
Shoulder stand
The Boat
The Bridge
The Lion
The Triangle
The Locust
The Bow
Cat stretch
Head-to-knee pose
Cat stretch
Head-to-knee pose
The Plow
The Cobra

Shavasana

Additional Notes

_____

_____

_____

_____

_____

_____

_____

_____

_____

_____

_____

_____

_____

_____

_____

_____

_____

_____

_____

Insight

Looking Further at Meditation Techniques

Because there are many different temperaments, there are many different meditative techniques. If you have never meditated you might wish to try several of the following techniques to discover which one will be the best for you. The main consideration is to be aware that this is a time to let go of your daily tensions and anxieties, a time to let your mind and body relax and just be. It is also a time to gain insights into your inner resources.

Witnessing

This is the purest form of meditation. It is simply sitting in meditation and watching the thoughts that come and go without judging or commenting. We are so caught up in our usual role of being absorbed with moment-to-moment thoughts that it is interesting to see what these thoughts consist of from a completely neutral position.

Listening

Meditation is centered in the idea of relaxing and non-doing. You may hear but you cannot listen when you are thinking. As you center your awareness in music, chanting, or natural sounds, you experience the essence of the sound, giving yourself the experience of emptiness, clarity, and receptivity.

Sound Current Meditation

Close your eyes and listen, with full attention, for whatever internal sound you may hear. If your thoughts intrude, do not be attached to them. Gradually, with practice and concentration, you will begin to hear a steady sound. It will seem to originate in your right ear. Keep your attention on the highest pitch that you can hear. Eventually, with practice, the sound will become centralized in the center of the brain and expanded until it includes the whole head. This sound is the aum vibration. Its source is the universal cosmic consciousness. Meditating on the sound current is considered to be one of the highest forms of meditation.

Meditation on the Light

The third eye center, or **ajna chakra** (Chapter 13), is located at the forehead. Close your eyes and concentrate on the point in back of the bridge of your nose while observing your inner field of vision. As you concentrate, a light will begin as a point of illumination and will expand until it includes your entire visual field. In the course of this practice you may begin to see the various chakras of the body, geometrical patterns, thought forms, scenery, and other visualizations.

In this meditation, as in the sound current meditation, it is important to become an observer. Thoughts or sounds come and go. Images present themselves, and the meditator observes them in much the same manner as one would passively watch a movie. In this way, the unconscious mind presents its own visual symbols before the conscious awareness, creating an automatic process of catharsis by which psychological problems are recognized, understood, and dismissed. Gradually this brings about an inner purification and produces a higher state of consciousness.

Meditation on the Breath (Vipassana)

Close your eyes and listen to the rhythm of your breath. This technique simply consists of observing the process of your breathing without trying to change or interfere with it. This practice eliminates distractions of the mind and emotions. It induces a quiet state in which deep levels of consciousness present themselves to conscious awareness. As you practice you will notice that the breathing naturally tends to become slow and rhythmic until it seems to pause of its own accord between breaths. All activity appears to be in a suspended state. Your body will breathe spontaneously when the demand for oxygen arises. This period of rest and quiet will purify and regenerate your entire body and mind.

Chapter 11

New Understandings:
Mantra Yoga

Asanas
Foot and Hand Pose (**Padahastasana**)
The Camel (**Ushtrasana**)

Insight:
Tratak (Gazing)

New Understandings
Mantra Yoga

In Sanskrit **man** is translated as "mind" and **tra** means "protection." Mantra yoga is a form of mental yoga in which the repetition of a sound evokes a deep reaction throughout the body. It can be practiced while sitting quietly in meditation, or at any time and place as a form of active meditation.

Mantras are energies that are thought to have existed always in the universe. They have passed for centuries in succession from teacher to disciple in an unbroken chain. As the energy of the mantra pervades your consciousness through constant repetition, it leads the way to meditation and to a state of oneness or nonduality.

On the physical level, many benefits are derived from **japa**, or repeating a mantra. For example, it can elicit a state of deep relaxation that revitalizes all of the cells and organs of your body. It also has a soothing and calming effect on the nervous system. Further benefits described by those who practice mantra yoga are an increase in concentration, a quieter mind, and a clearing of anger, worry, anxiety, and fear.

There are two main types of mantras, deity and vedantic. A **deity mantra** is one that evokes a particular deity and concentrates on the qualities of the deity. The following are examples of deity mantras.

Shiva: **Om namah Shivaya**.

Shiva is said to be the Lord of Auspiciousness, and the representation of the universal power of destruction in which all existence ends and from which it arises again. The repetition of **om/na/mah/shi/va/ya** should be done slowly, timing the phrasing with each inhalation and each exhalation.

Vishnu: **Om nama Narayanaya** (Vishnu is also called Narayan).

Lord Vishnu is thought to be the preserver of the universe, and embodies the qualities of mercy, goodness, and the all-pervading power which preserves and maintains the universe and the cosmic order. As in **om namah Shivaya**, repeat **om/namo/nar/a/yan/aya** with each inhalation and each exhalation of your breath.

Vedantic mantras are more abstract and relate to pure sound or energy. Two examples of vedantic mantras are below.

Om: This is thought to be the original mantra. In the Bible it says, "In the beginning was the word and the word was with God and the word was God." In Indian philosophies, om is thought to have been the first vibration of sound from which all other sounds emerged. It is used at the beginning and end of all prayers in the yogic tradition just as amen, which carries the same vibration, concludes all prayers in the Christian tradition. Repeating this mantra with complete concentration on its sound and meaning is considered to be an extremely effective spiritual practice. The repetition is done very slowly with a sustained humming resonance that you will find soothing and relaxing. Coordinate the mantra with your breath, and attempt to strengthen your inhalations and exhalations as you practice.

Ham-sa or **so-ham** (**so-hum**): This means "I am that" or "I am he." This mantra represents a remembrance of the fact that there is no real difference between the self whom we identify ourselves to be and the higher or universal self. When you practice the mantra, emphasize the resonance or the humming sound of ham or hum as you inhale slowly. As you slowly exhale, focus your attention on lengthening the sound of sa. In this meditation your focus will eventually be brought to the space between breaths. This is the goal of all meditation, to become aware of and in balance with the space of the higher self, which is thought to exist in the quiet place between breaths and also in the space between two thoughts.

Symbol of Om

Foot and Hand Pose

(Padahastasana)
(Pada, foot; hasta, hand)

Benefits
Stretches the hamstring muscles, provides a lateral stretch to the spine, and trims the waistline.

Basic position
Stand straight with your feet wide apart. Clasp your hands behind your back.

Instructions
Twist your upper body to the left and bend toward your left foot.
Bring your hands to your ankle and your forehead as close to your foot as you can.
You may have to bend your left knee slightly to assume this position.
Hold between five and ten counts.
Slowly return to your original position and repeat on the other side.
Practice three to five times on each side.

Breathing
Inhale while standing erect.
Exhale while bending.
Breathe normally while stretching.
Inhale while returning to your original position.

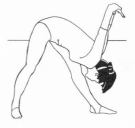

CHART YOUR PROGRESS - Degree of difficulty

Date	Hard 1	2	3	4	5	6	7	Easy 8	Date	Hard 1	2	3	4	5	6	7	Easy 8

Chart Your Progress
Body Awareness

Foot and Hand Pose

Date

The Camel

(Ushtrasana)
(Ushtra: camel)

Benefits
Aids the digestion and elimination, and strengthens the lower back, arms, and legs.

Basic position
Kneel on the floor, knees and feet a shoulder-width apart, arms at your sides.

Instructions
Carefully arch your back, and place your right hand on your right heel and your left hand on your left heel.
Arch your head back and press your hips forward.
Contract your buttocks muscles and keep the weight of your body over your knees.
Remain in the stretch as long as you comfortably can.
Slowly return to the basic position.
Repeat up to five times.
After your last stretch (to avoid back problems), lie on your back and hug your knees to your chest for a full minute.

Breathing
Inhale while in the basic position.
Exhale while bending backwards.
Breathe normally while in the stretch.
Exhale while returning to the basic position.

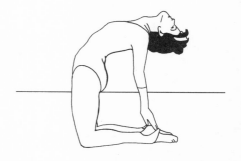

CHART YOUR PROGRESS - Degree of difficulty																
	Hard						Easy		Hard							Easy
Date	1	2	3	4	5	6	7	8	Date	1	2	3	4	5	6	7	8

Chart Your Progress
Body Awareness

The Camel

Date
_____

_____

_____

_____

_____

_____

_____

_____

_____

_____

_____

_____

_____

_____

_____

_____

_____

Your Progam

Warm-ups
Sun salutation
Head rolls
Shoulder rotations
Foot exercises
Shoulder clasp
Spinal rock
The Butterfly

Breathing exercises
Complete breath
Choose additional breathing
  exercises as desired.

Asanas
Double angle pose
The Fish
Foot-balancing pose
Upright head-to-knee pose
Leg pulls
Shoulder stand
The Boat
The Bridge
The Lion
The Triangle
The Locust
The Bow
Cat stretch
Head-to-knee pose
Cat stretch
Head-to-knee pose
The Plow
The Cobra
Foot and hand pose
The Camel

Shavasana

Additional Notes

Insight
Tratak (Gazing)

The state of no thought or quiet mind is the ultimate state sought by the yoga student. It has been called the state of pure consciousness or unconditioned knowledge. It is characterized in metaphysical literature as supreme enlightenment that transcends anything known through external vision.

Three simple gazing techniques will give you the experience of quiet mind within a relatively short time: candle gazing, mandala contemplation, and yantra.

Candle Gazing

Candle gazing is a well-known method to provide the seed for meditation. The flame is classic in its ability to provide the impetus for a deep state of meditation. It is restful for the eyes, and the impression it makes on the retina is relatively simple to retain.

Place a lighted candle three or four feet from you. Sit in a meditation posture and start to control your breath gently as you gaze at the flame of the candle. As you gaze, become aware only of the flame, noting its shape, movement, and color. After you have studied this with a clear gaze for several minutes, close your eyes (cup your hands over your eyes, if you wish). See the flame of the candle in your mind's eye and quietly maintain the image. When it finally fades, open your eyes. You can repeat the pattern two or three times. The more you practice the more adept you will become.

Mandala Contemplation

Mandala contemplation, in which the meditator loses all thought of immediate needs or wishes, is an ancient technique for stilling the mind. A mandala is a rather large and intricate design in which the entire pattern leads you ultimately to focus on the center. Gazing at a mandala for ten minutes or more helps you to center your thoughts and to bring you to a point of single-minded concentration. Mandalas can be purchased at many metaphysical bookstores. It is important to choose one that is pleasing to you personally in both design and color.

Yantra

A yantra is a visual symbol. It can be very simple such as a circle or a triangle, or much more complicated and elaborate. All yantras are universal symbols. They are used as seeds for meditation not only in yoga, but, with various
modifications, in esoteric practices throughout the world. Each yantra imparts
its own individual form of energy and vibration.

The combination of a yantra and its related mantra is a powerful meditation practice. The energy it generates has a lasting effect and produces a quality of positiveness and elevated consciousness that continues long after
meditation has ended. It is considered by many advanced students of yoga to
be the ultimate meditation. For your practice, the om mantra-yantra has been
included here. A number of excellent books are available on the subject
should you wish to practice this technique with other yantras.

Sit in a meditation posture with your eyes open. Place the symbol
(found on page 136) where you can see it comfortably without lowering your head. Hold your gaze steadily on the figure for several minutes, and simultaneously perform audible intonations of om. Breathe
deeply and normally.

Your attention can alternate between the figure and the sound.
Eventually, they will merge, and your attention will be focused on that
point of merge. After several minutes have elapsed, close your eyes and
visualize the om symbol. Simultaneously, without interrupting the
rhythm you have established for the audible intonations, continue with
silent repetitions of om.

If you lose the mental image, open your eyes and concentrate for several more minutes before your next visualization. Continue practicing
this mantra-yantra combination until your meditation becomes
smooth and flowing.

Chapter 12

New Understandings:
A Beautiful You Through Better Eating

Asanas
Spinal Twist (**Ardha Matsyendrasana**)
Half Lotus (**Ardha Padmasana**)

Insight:
Balancing Food, Balancing You

New Understandings
A More Beautiful You Through Better Eating

In Chapter 3, you learned that **prana** is defined in Sanskrit as the life force that is essential to sustain every living thing. Food is one of the important sources of **prana**. The other sources are air, sleep, water, and sunlight.

When foods are processed by any means, the life force of the original substance becomes depleted. Foods that cannot be properly digested or quickly eliminated may contribute to many illnesses because they encourage a build-up of excess toxins and waste products.

The typical American diet of highly processed foods containing large amounts of fats, sugars, and starches can decrease vitality and endurance. Since what you eat has a pronounced effect on how you feel and act, all foods should be consumed in as natural a state as possible. It is necessary to think about eating, not simply to satisfy desires, but to increase your store of energy. Foods high in life force help to regenerate your body, whereas devitalized foods can sap your vitality and cause the symptoms of aging. When your body is in a pure, clean, healthy state and filled with a maximum of life force, it has a greater capacity to heal itself and function with vibrant health and energy.

The following suggestions and guidelines will enable you to develop the habit of selecting the proper foods for maintaining a high level of vitality.

Do not eat overcooked foods. Eat an abundance of raw fruits and raw or lightly cooked vegetables in season. Use tree-ripened fruits and garden-ripened vegetables whenever possible. Choose a wide variety of natural foods, to avoid a repetitious diet. Avoid artificial foods and beverages, canned foods, and foods that are fried or cooked in deep fat. Avoid foods containing white flour and white sugar. Avoid products containing artificial stimulants such as coffee, alcohol, and caffeine (black tea, chocolate, some soft drinks). Also avoid highly processed foods such as candies, cakes, pastry, and most dry cereals.

Purchase only dairy products containing a low amount of fat. Lean red meat should be consumed moderately; poultry and fish are better choices. Bake, broil, or steam meats whenever possible, being sure to trim off all visible fat. Meals should be light and fully nourishing. All foods should be eaten slowly and chewed well.

Spinal Twist

(Ardha Matsyendrasana)
(Ardha, half; matsyendra, sage)

Benefits

Increases back and spine flexibility, tones the spinal nerves, massages internal organs, slims the waistline, and strengthens the leg muscles.

Basic position

Sit on the floor with your legs outstretched.

Instructions

Place your right foot on the floor on the outside of your left knee.
Bend your left leg to the right and bring your left heel against the right buttock.
Sit as straight as you can and slowly turn your upper body to the right.
Bring your left hand around the outside of your right knee and hold onto your right ankle.
Attempt to place your right knee close to your left armpit.
Place your right hand behind your back and look over your right shoulder.
Hold the pose as long as you comfortably can.
Slowly return to the basic position.
Change legs and repeat on the other side.
Repeat two or three times to each side.

Breathing

Exhale while twisting.
Breathe normally while in the posture.
Inhale while returning to the basic position.

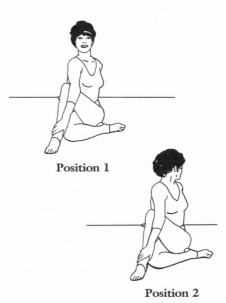

Position 1

Position 2

Caution

It is important to move gently in and out of a twist. To avoid overstretching, twist only to a degree of comfort. Avoid straining. Gradually increase the twist as the muscles and vertebrae become more flexible. Until the necessary flexibility has been acquired, practice this asana with your lower leg outstretched and your free hand touching the floor behind you for balance.

CHART YOUR PROGRESS - Degree of difficulty

	Hard							Easy		Hard							Easy
Date	1	2	3	4	5	6	7	8	Date	1	2	3	4	5	6	7	8

Chart Your Progress
Body Awareness

Spinal Twist

Date

Half Lotus Pose

(Ardha Padmasana)
(Ardha, half; padma, lotus)

Benefits
The half lotus posture is a meditative pose in which one can maintain steadiness in a seated position for a long period of time.
Steadiness of the body brings steadiness of the mind which is the first step toward productive meditation.

Basic position
Sit with your legs extended forward.

Instructions
Place your left foot next to your right thigh.
Draw your right foot to the top of your left thigh or as high on the left leg as you comfortably can place it. Keep your back and head as straight as possible. By alternately placing each foot in the elevated position, you will gradually be able to attain the full lotus posture.

Limitations
Do not do the full posture if you have sciatica or lower back problems. Use a cross legged position instead.

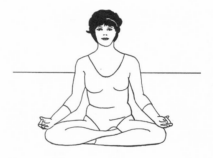

CHART YOUR PROGRESS - Degree of difficulty																	
	Hard						Easy			Hard							Easy
Date	1	2	3	4	5	6	7	8	Date	1	2	3	4	5	6	7	8

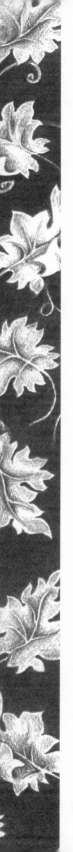

Chart Your Progress
Body Awareness

Half Lotus Pose

Date

Your Progam

Warm-ups
Sun salutation
Head rolls
Shoulder rotations
Foot exercises
Shoulder clasp
Spinal rock
The Butterfly

Breathing exercises
Complete breath
Choose additional breathing
  exercises as desired.

Asanas
Double angle pose
The Fish
Foot-balancing pose
Upright head-to-knee pose
Leg pulls
Shoulder stand
The Boat
The Bridge
The Lion
The Triangle
The Locust
The Bow
Cat stretch
Head-to-knee pose
The Plow
The Cobra
Foot and hand pose
The Camel
Spinal twist
Half lotus

Shavasana

Additional Notes

_____

_____

_____

_____

_____

_____

_____

_____

_____

_____

_____

_____

_____

_____

_____

_____

_____

Insight
Balancing Food, Balancing You

The principle of yin and yang is known as the Unifying Principle because it states that antagonistic forces complement and unify each other. In yogic philosophy there is nothing but yin and yang in the relative world. All manifestations are seen as a blending of these two opposites and choosing to eat foods that compliment each other is considered to be the best way to remain balanced and whole. Eating a diet that is too yin is thought to disperse life force while foods that are too yang are believed to stifle energy and well-being. It is also felt that either extreme creates disease and unhappiness while foods that contain an equal amount of yin and yang create harmony.

The basic characteristics of a food determine whether it is yin or yang. This takes into account the different factors in the growth and structure of foods.

Characteristics of Yin Foods
>   Growth in a hot climate or in summer
>   More rapid growth
>   Foods containing more water
>   Fruits and leaves
>   Major growth above the ground
>   Sour, bitter, sharply sweet, hot, and aromatic foods

Characteristics of Yang Foods
>   Growth in a cold climate or in winter
>   Slower growth
>   Drier foods
>   Stems, roots, and seeds
>   Major growth below the ground
>   Salty, plainly sweet, and pungent foods

Yang — Contracting Energy
> Strong Yang Foods
>   Refined salt
>   Eggs
>   Meat
>   Cheese
>   Poultry
>   Fatty fish
>   Seafood

More Balanced Foods

Whole cereal grains

Beans and bean products

Roots, round, and leafy green vegetables

Sea vegetables

Unrefined sea salt, vegetable oil, and other seasonings

Spring water

Non-aromatic, non-stimulant teas and beverages

Seeds and nuts

Temperate climate fruit

Rice syrup, barley malt, and other grain-based natural sweeteners (used in moderation)

Yin — Expanding Energy

Strong Yin Foods

White rice, white flour

Frozen and canned foods

Tropical fruits and vegetables

Milk, cream, yogurt, and ice cream

Refined oils

Spices (pepper, curry, nutmeg, etc.)

Aromatic and stimulant beverages (coffee, black tea, mint tea, etc.)

Honey, sugar, and refined sweeteners

Most Western diets combine foods from the strong yang category and the strong yin category. According to the yogic way of eating, food out of harmony with our bodily needs, such as meats, eggs and hard salty cheeses, which are all yang, stimulate a craving for opposite, or yin, foods such as sugar, coffee, alcohol, ice cream and tropical fruits. The swings from one extreme to the other are thought to destroy the body's balance and deplete its energy which in turn leads to illness and fatigue.

Chapter 13

New Understandings:
Yogic Power Centers: The **Chakras**

Asanas
The Wheel Pose (**Chakrasana**)
Back Stretch (**Paschimottanasana**)

Insight:
Slow Motion

New Understandings
Yogic Power Centers: The Chakras

As we have seen in Chapter 5, the symbol for yin and yang represents the laws of change and the dynamic curve dividing them suggests that they are continuously merging. The small circles of opposite shading illustrate that a part of yin must remain yang and a part of yang must remain yin. Thus, yin and yang create each other, transform into each other, and depend upon each other for definition. Because they are continually contracting and expanding, the yogic tradition supports the belief that this movement is the source of the energy that animates all living things.

Throughout the ages the image of energy flowing through the body has been a part of the basic symbolism of healing. In China it is the **chi** energy in t'ai chi. In India it is called **prana**. This energy is thought to flow from seven circles of light or energy sources called **chakras**. (In Sanskrit **chakra** means "wheel.") The seven **chakras** relate to the major nerve plexuses and endocrine glands in the physical body. These are the main control centers in the body and the asanas of hatha yoga have a beneficial effect on one or more of these plexuses. For example, the Shoulder Stand exerts a strong pressure on the thyroid gland in the throat, which is associated with the fifth chakra. The thyroid is given greater stimulation and improved function results when concentration is also focused on this area during the asana.

Chart of the Seven Chakras

NAME: First **chakra**, BASE CENTER
      Mooladhara (**mool**—root, **adhara**—place)
LOCATION: Base of the spine
ENDOCRINE INFLUENCE: Ovaries, gonads
COLOR: Red

NAME: Second **chakra,** SPLEEN CENTER
      Swadhistana chakra (**swa**—self, **sthan**—dwelling place)
LOCATION: Halfway between pubis and navel
ENDOCRINE INFLUENCE: liver, pancreas, spleen
COLOR: Orange

NAME: Third **chakra**, SOLAR PLEXUS
    Manipura chakra (**mani**—jewel, **pura**—city)
LOCATION: Slightly above the navel
ENDOCRINE INFLUENCE: Adrenal glands
COLOR: Yellow

NAME: Fourth **chakra**, HEART CENTER
    Anahata chakra (**an**—not, **ahat**—struck)
LOCATION: Center of the chest
ENDOCRINE INFLUENCE: Thymus gland
COLOR: Green

NAME: Fifth **chakra**, THROAT CENTER
    Vishuddhi chakra (**vishuddhi**—to purify)
LOCATION: Middle of the throat
ENDOCRINE INFLUENCE: Thyroid gland
COLOR: Blue

NAME: Sixth **chakra**, BROW CENTER
    Ajna chakra (**ajna**—to command)
LOCATION: Middle of the forehead
ENDOCRINE INFLUENCE: Pineal gland
COLOR: Indigo

NAME: Seventh **chakra**, CROWN CENTER
    Bindu chakra (**bindu**—a point or a drop)
LOCATION: Top of the head
ENDOCRINE INFLUENCE: Pituitary gland
COLOR: Violet

Chakra Exercise

The following exercises will give you a greater understanding of each of the seven **chakras**. You will be able to locate, and balance, the level of energy in each **chakra**. When your energy levels are high and thoroughly balanced you will notice a sense of well-being and energy throughout your entire body. This exercise should be done with a partner. You will need a lightly weighted chain or pendulum.

Exercise 1:

Lie comfortably on your back. Take several deep breaths and relax as much as possible. Starting at the base **chakra**, have the person you are working with hold the weight approximately three inches from the surface of your body. The hand holding the thread or chain must be relaxed and still. Your partner's energy plus the energy from the **chakra** will soon cause the weight to move. If the weight moves in a clockwise circle, the **chakra** is energized and balanced. If the weight moves in any other way or does not move at all, close your eyes and visualize the color of the **chakra** for approximately three minutes. Repeat the exercise until the energy is flowing smoothly in a clockwise circle.

Exercise 2:

Lie comfortably on your back. Take several deep breaths and relax as much as possible. Place your hands over each **chakra** in succession (starting with the first **chakra**), for at least three minutes. Visualize the color of the **chakra** moving in a clockwise circle around and through the **chakra**. If you find it difficult to visualize the circling energy, use your hands to draw a slow circle as you visualize the color. If you find it difficult to visualize the color just repeat the word for the color as you do the exercise.

Once you have started either of these exercises, you should balance the energy equally in all seven **chakras**.

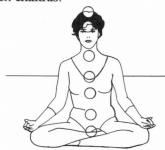

The Wheel

(Chakrasana)
(Chakra, wheel)

Benefits
Strengthens back and arm muscles, tones arms, legs, waist and spine, reverses blood flow, and aids in digestion and elimination.

Basic position
Lie on your back with your knees bent and your heels close to your buttocks. Arms comfortably at your sides.

Instructions
Bend your arms with elbows pointing toward the ceiling.
Place your fingertips underneath your shoulders.
Slowly raise your body in a straight line from your knees to your shoulders.
Using the strength of your arms, raise your shoulders off the floor and let the crown of your head rest on the floor to support the weight of your upper body.
Straighten your arms and legs, lift your head off the floor and raise your body to a fully arched height.
Remain in the position as long as you comfortably can.
Slowly lower your body back to the head-based, then the supine position.
Practice the Wheel one time for as long as you can comfortably hold the posture.
After your stretch (to avoid back problems), lie on your back and hug your knees for a full minute.

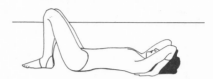

Position 1

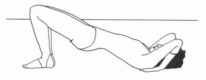

Position 2

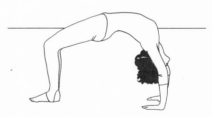

Position 3

Breathing

Inhale as you begin the stretch.
Retain the breath inside as you hold the posture.
Exhale as you return to the starting position.
After regular practice, the posture may be maintained for longer periods by breathing normally in the fully extended position.

Limitations

Do not practice The Wheel if you have high blood pressure, ulcers, heart problems, lower back pain, or if you have recently fractured a bone or had surgery. If you are a beginner you should first concentrate on the easier backward bending asanas. If you cannot maintain the full stretch, use the intermediate position, with head support, until your back becomes stronger and more flexible.

CHART YOUR PROGRESS - Degree of difficulty

	Hard							Easy		Hard							Easy
Date	1	2	3	4	5	6	7	8	Date	1	2	3	4	5	6	7	8

160

Chart Your Progress
Body Awareness

The Wheel

Date

The Back Stretch

(Paschimottanasana)
(Paschimottana, whole body; asana, stretch)

Benefits
Stretches the hamstring muscles, loosens the hip joints, tones the abdominal organs and muscles, tones the pelvic organs, and encourages blood to flow to the spinal nerves and muscles.

Basic position
Sit on the floor with your legs straight in front of you.
Rest your hands on your thighs.

Instructions
Consciously relax your whole body.
Relax your back and stomach muscles and slowly bend forward, sliding your hands along the top of your legs.
Hold your feet or ankles and consciously relax your back and leg muscles.
Keep your legs straight and, using only your arms, pull your upper body forward toward your legs. This should be a gentle process without any sudden movement or excessive strain.
If possible touch your forehead to your knees and hold onto your toes.
If you are a beginner, stretch as far as you can without straining.
Remain in the final pose for a comfortable length of time and then slowly return to the starting position.
Repeat three or four times.

Breathing
Inhale before you start.
Exhale slowly while bending forward.
Inhale while holding the stretch.
Exhale as you stretch farther forward.
Breathe slowly and deeply in the final posture.
Inhale slowly while returning to the starting position.

Limitations
You should not do this asana if you have lower back pain, sciatica, or chronic arthritis.

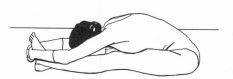

CHART YOUR PROGRESS - Degree of difficulty																	
	Hard						Easy		Hard							Easy	
Date	1	2	3	4	5	6	7	8	Date	1	2	3	4	5	6	7	8

Chart Your Progress
Body Awareness

The Back Stretch

Date

_____

_____

_____

_____

_____

_____

_____

_____

_____

_____

_____

_____

_____

_____

_____

_____

_____

Your Program

Warm-ups
Sun salutation
Head rolls
Shoulder rotations
Foot exercises
Shoulder clasp
Spinal rock
The Butterfly

Breathing exercises
Complete breath
Choose additional breathing
 exercises as desired.

Asanas
Double angle pose
The Fish
Foot-balancing pose
Upright head-to-knee pose
Leg pulls
Shoulder stand
The Boat
The Bridge
The Lion
The Triangle
The Locust
The Bow
Cat stretch
Head-to-knee pose
The Plow
The Cobra
Foot and hand pose
The Camel
Spinal twist
Half lotus
The Wheel
Back stretch

Shavasana

Additional Notes

Insight
Slow Motion

Focus on an everyday task such as eating, getting dressed, combing your hair, or preparing for bed. Do it at half speed while paying close attention to how your body feels. Be aware of body movement, tensions, or feelings of discomfort. Let yourself feel what your body is experiencing.

Take a moment to describe any new feelings or body sensations that you have not previously noticed. If you find, for example, that you are holding tension in any area of your body you can then begin to relax that tension.

Since it takes an enormous amount of energy to hold muscles in a semi-contracted state, you will have a more complete energy balance when you begin to recognize and release held stresses and tensions.

Chapter 14

New Understandings:
Your Energy Field: Your Aura

Asanas
Spiraled Head-to-Knee Pose (**Parivritti Janusirshasana**)
Head Stand (**Sirshasana**)

Insight:
Imagining Yourself

New Understandings:

Your Energy Field: Your Aura

Researchers working with Kirlian photography have demonstrated that the energy field or colored, light area surrounding the human body can be seen as seven layers of light. Changes in these electro-magnetic fields have long been thought to be related to health and disease. Two major aims of yoga are to balance and clear the **chakras** and to clear the aura of dark or "unhealthy" colors. Just as the energy flow through the **chakras** is thought to bring optimum health when they are opened, the energy field outside the human body (which is the sum total of the energy given off by the **chakras**) relates to overall biological functioning.

Aura Exercises

Sit as straight as you can in a cross legged or half lotus position.

Exercise 1.

Clap your hands for about 30 seconds.

Place them, palms up, on your knees.

Close your eyes and experience the feeling in your hands.

You will feel the stinging on the surface.

Let it flow up your arms and around your body. Enjoy experiencing the energy flow in a detached way.

Exercise 2.

Sit with your eyes closed.

Place your hands in front of you with your palms facing each other (about two or three inches apart).

Move them closer and farther apart.

After awhile you will become aware of a feeling of resistance between your hands.

Exercise 3.

Sit with your eyes closed.

Imagine that you are holding a warm ball of energy.

After you have felt a change in the temperature in your hands, let the heat travel wherever it will around or through your body.

Exercise 4.

Close your eyes and imagine glowing pink light at the level of your heart.

Hold it there for a slow count of 9.

Move the light to a space just above the top of your head.

Hold it there for a slow count of 18.

Visualize a pink light surrounding your entire body.

Sit in the center of the light for a slow count of 20.

Next, create a blue light at the level of your throat.

Hold it there for a slow count of 9.

Move the light to a space just above the top of your head.

Hold it there for a slow count of 18.

Visualize a blue light surrounding your entire body.

Sit in the center of the light for a slow count 20.

Next, create a white light at the level of your forehead.

Hold it there for a slow count of 9.

Move the light to a space just above your head. Hold it there for a slow count of 18.

Visualize a white light surrounding your entire body.

Sit in the center of the light for a slow count of 20.

Slowly open your eyes and experience how you feel.

This process can relax and energize your entire body.

Exercise 5.

Sit facing a partner with your eyes open. Rub or clap your hands for about 30 seconds.

Extend the palms of your hands toward the open palms of your partner who is seated facing you with closed eyes.

Rotate your hands in a clockwise circle for two minutes.

Ask your partner if there is a change in sensation or if the rotation movement can be felt.

You may also move your hands back and forth or up and down.

Ask your partner to describe the different sensations.

Exercise 6.

To see an aura:

Place a chair in front of a mirror which shows your reflection against a plain background.

Decrease the lighting in the room so that it resembles dusk.

Sit comfortably in your chair and pick out a spot about six inches above your head and two feet behind you.

As you stare at that spot, within five minutes you will become aware of an outline, seen peripherally, around your head and shoulders.

If you practice for five minutes each morning and evening, within a few days you will begin to see an outline aura extending one to two feet.

With continued practice the details of color and shade will be added to what you have learned to perceive.

Eventually you will be able to experience seeing auras at any time and in any light.

This exercise can also be practiced with a partner.

Spiraled Head-to-Knee Pose
(Parivritti Janusirshasana)
(Parivritti, spiraled; janu, knee; sirsa, head)

Benefits
Tones the spinal nerves, and strengthens the back, abdomen, and chest.

Basic position
Sit on the floor with your legs straight in front of you.

Instructions
Bend your left leg and place the heel against your thigh.
Stretch to the right and hold your right foot with your right hand.
Your fingers should be in contact with the instep and your palm should be turned upward.
Place your elbow on the inside of your right leg.
Twist your body as much as you comfortably can without straining.
Bring your left arm over your head and hold the toes of your right foot.
If you cannot reach your foot, hold onto your leg.
Stretch your left arm over your head and sideways as far as you can without straining.
Stay in the asana a comfortable length of time.
Slowly return to your original position.
Repeat to the other side.
Repeat three or four times on each side.

Breathing
Inhale before you start.
Exhale while stretching to the side.
Breathe normally while in the posture.
Inhale while returning to the basic position.

Limitations
Do not do this stretch if you have lower back problems or if you are pregnant.

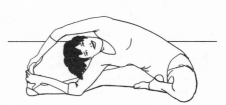

CHART YOUR PROGRESS - Degree of difficulty																	
	Hard						Easy			Hard							Easy
Date	1	2	3	4	5	6	7	8	Date	1	2	3	4	5	6	7	8

Chart Your Progress
Body Awareness

Spiraled Head-to-Knee Pose

Date

_____

_____

_____

_____

_____

_____

_____

_____

_____

_____

_____

_____

_____

_____

_____

_____

Head Stand

(Sirshasana)
(Sirsa, head)

Benefits
Increases the blood flow to the brain, reverses the upward return flow of blood in the legs and viscera, and revitalizes the mind and body.

Basic position
Kneel on the floor with your back straight and arms at your sides.

Instructions
Bend forward and place your forearms on the floor, with your fingers intertwined and your elbows in front of your knees.
Place the crown of your head between your hands.
Be sure that your head is firmly supported.
Straighten your legs and raise your buttocks.
Slowly walk your legs toward your trunk. Allow your knees to bend so that your back is upright.
Slowly transfer your body weight from your toes onto your head and arms.
Raise one foot a few inches off the ground.
Raise the other foot and balance on your head and arms.
When you feel that you have your balance, raise and straighten your hips so that your thighs move up and away from your body.
Slowly straighten your legs. Your body should be perfectly straight in the final posture.
If you are a beginner it is helpful to have someone hold your back and feet to help you gain confidence.
Hold the posture as long as you are comfortable.
Gently return to the basic position.
After a short rest, repeat up to three times.

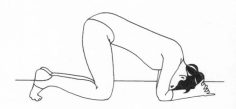

Position 1

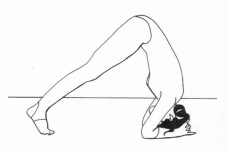

Position 2

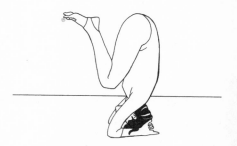

Position 3

Breathing
Take a deep breath and hold your breath inside while assuming and returning from the asana.
Breathe normally once your balance has been obtained.

Limitation
Do not do the head stand if you have high blood pressure.

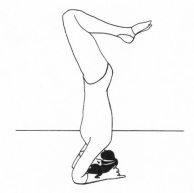

Position 4

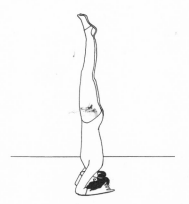

Position 5

CHART YOUR PROGRESS - Degree of difficulty

	Hard							Easy		Hard							Easy
Date	1	2	3	4	5	6	7	8	Date	1	2	3	4	5	6	7	8

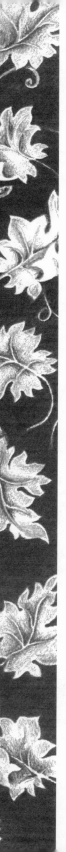

Chart Your Progress
Body Awareness

Head Stand

Date

_____

_____

_____

_____

_____

_____

_____

_____

_____

_____

_____

_____

_____

_____

_____

_____

_____

_____

Your Program

Warm-ups
Sun salutation
Head rolls
Shoulder rotations
Foot exercises
Shoulder clasp
Spinal rock
The Butterfly

Breathing exercises
Complete breath
Choose additional breathing
  exercises as desired.

Asanas
Double angle pose
The Fish
Foot-balancing pose
Upright head-to-knee pose
Leg pulls
Shoulder stand
The Boat
The Bridge
The Lion
The Triangle
The Locust
The Bow
Cat stretch
Head-to-knee pose
The Plow
The Cobra
Foot and hand pose
The Camel
Spinal twist
Half lotus
The Wheel
Back stretch
Spiral head-to-knee pose
Head stand

Shavasana

Additional Notes

Insight
Imagining Yourself

Visualization allows you to take a mini-vacation whenever and wherever you wish. Sit quietly with your eyes closed and evoke an image of your favorite place, flower, or other special feature or item. With practice you will be able to enjoy the details of your projection as clearly as if it were placed before you in real life. As you concentrate, your visualization can become so lifelike that you might imagine the fragrance of a flower or hear the sounds that you would expect to hear in your special place.

Spend at least five minutes at a time evoking the image. When you have finished, take a moment to write a brief description of your visualization. Include any sensations of deeper relaxation or increased awareness that you experienced.

Chapter 15

New Understandings:
Putting It All Together

Asanas

The Crane (**Bakasana**)

King of Dancer's Pose I (**Natarajasana I**)

King of Dancer's Pose II (**Natarajasana II**)

One-Leg Stand (**Eka Padasana**)

Tree Pose (**Vrikshasana**)

Half-Moon Pose(**Ardha Chandrasana**)

Palm Tree Pose (**Talasana**)

The Peacock (**Mayurasana**)

Insight:
Further Your Self-Discovery

New Understandings
Putting It All Together

Now that your program has become well established, you may wish to practice several more difficult asanas. The postures in this chapter will help you to gain even more balance and control, and will add an extra challenge. As you continue to attain strength and flexibility, you may wish to incorporate one or more of these postures into your daily practice.

Your future goals may also include an interest in strengthening specific body areas. Therefore, this chapter contains a chart listing asanas that will help you to become strong and flexible where needed. To personalize your program, you may wish to spend extra time working with the asanas that will best benefit your individual needs.

This journal is meant to aid you in your constant process of growth and change. As you continue to practice, use the extra page after each asana to chart your progress.

It would also be helpful to keep a record of changes in your diet, sleeping habits, or relaxation patterns, and any other changes that you are now incorporating into your daily life. In the back of the book you will find a section in which you can record your current new understandings, your further progress, and notes of interest.

It is my hope that you will continue your yoga practice for a lifetime of health and well-being, and that you share your skills with others. You have by now discovered that you can expect many new and valuable changes in your mind, body, and spirit from spending just a short time each day with the material presented in this book. Your ability to personalize a system that has been in existence for over two thousand years allows you to transform these special techniques for your own use, and to send this energy out in your own way to affect the world around you.

Exercises for Specific Areas

Abdomen: The Plow
The Bow
The Locust
The Cobra
Shoulder stand
The Boat

Back and Spine:
The Plow
The Locust
The Bow
Leg pulls
Spinal twist
The Fish
The Bridge
Head-to-toe pose
The Wheel
Back stretch
Spinal rock
(warm-ups)

Balance: All of the postures
in Chapter 15
Heel raises

Bust and Chest:
Shoulder clasp
(warm-ups)
The Triangle
The Bow
The Cobra
Double angle pose
The Fish
Head-to-toe pose
The Wheel

Arms, Hands, and Shoulders:
Cat stretch
The Wheel
The Cobra
Double angle pose

Feet: Half lotus
Heel raises
Leg pulls
The Bridge
The Wheel
The Butterfly
(warm-ups)

Hips: The Locust
The Boat
Leg pulls
All of the postures

Neck: Head rolls
Double angle pose
The Fish
The Cobra
The Plow
Cat stretch
Shoulder stand
The Wheel

Shoulders: The Plow
Shoulder clasp
(warm-ups)
Double angle pose
The Wheel
The Cobra
Shoulder stand
Head stand

Buttocks:	The Locust	**Circulation:**	All of the postures in
	The Cobra		Chapter 15
	Shoulder stand		Head stand
	The Plow		Shoulder stand
	The Bow		The Plow
	Alternate leg pull		The Bridge
	The Bridge		Head-to-knee pose
			Spiral head-to-knee
Face:	The Lion		pose
	Double angle pose		
	Head-to-knee pose	**Thighs:**	The Triangle
	Head-to-toe pose		The Butterfly
	Spiral head-to-knee		The Locust
	pose		The Bow
	Shoulder stand		The Camel
	The Plow		The Wheel
	The Wheel		

The Crane

(Bakasana)
(Baka, crane)

Benefits
Improves blood circulation to the brain, and strengthens the arms, shoulders, and leg muscles.

Basic position
Stand erect with your feet together and your arms raised about your head.

Instructions
Bend at the waist and hold onto your left foot or ankle with both hands.
At the same time stretch your right leg up and back as high as you can.
Keep your knees as straight as possible and hold the position as long as you wish.
Lower your leg and slowly return to the standing position.
Repeat on the other side.
Practice the asana three times to each side.

Breathing
Inhale while raising your arms.
Exhale while bending forward.
Breathe normally while in the final posture.
Inhale while returning to the standing position.

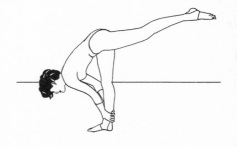

CHART YOUR PROGRESS - Degree of difficulty																	
	Hard							Easy		Hard							Easy
Date	1	2	3	4	5	6	7	8	Date	1	2	3	4	5	6	7	8

Chart Your Progress
Body Awareness

The Crane

Date

_____

_____

_____

_____

_____

_____

_____

_____

_____

_____

_____

_____

_____

_____

_____

_____

_____

_____

King of Dancer's Pose
(Natarajasana I)
(Nataraja, king of dancers)

Benefits
Balances the nervous system, aids in bodily control and mental concentration, and strengthens the back, legs, and hips.

Basic position
Stand with your feet a shoulder-width apart.
Be sure your weight is distributed evenly and your arms are relaxed at your sides.

Instructions
Focus your eyes on a specific point in front of you, while keeping your head straight.
Raise your left foot and reach back with your left hand to grasp the foot firmly.
Raise your right arm.
Try to maintain your balance.
Continue stretching upward as you hold the position.
Hold the position as long as you wish.
Slowly return to the original position.
Change legs and repeat.
Do the asana three times on each side.

Breathing
Inhale while bringing your arm and leg together.
Breathe normally while in the posture.
Inhale while returning to the starting position.

Limitations
If you have a weak stomach or back muscles, you should not attempt this exercise until you first strengthen these muscles with other asanas.

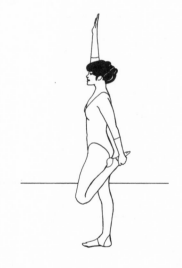

CHART YOUR PROGRESS - Degree of difficulty																	
	Hard							Easy		Hard							Easy
Date	1	2	3	4	5	6	7	8	Date	1	2	3	4	5	6	7	8

Chart Your Progress
Body Awareness

King of Dancer's Pose I

Date

King of Dancer's Pose II
(Natarajasana II)

Benefits
Balances the nervous system, aids in balance and mental concentration, and builds strong legs and hips.

Basic position
Stand with your feet a shoulder-width apart.
Be sure your weight is distributed evenly and your arms are relaxed at your sides.

Instructions
Bend your left leg backward and raise your left foot as high as possible.
Grasp the left ankle with the left hand.
Reach upward and forward with the right arm and look at your right hand.
Continue stretching upward as you hold the position.
Hold the posture as long as you comfortably can.
Slowly return to the original position.
Change legs and repeat.
Do the asana three times on each side.

Breathing
Inhale while establishing the position.
Breathe normally while in the posture.
Inhale while returning to the starting position.

Limitations
If you have a weak stomach or back muscles, you should not do this exercise until you first strengthen these muscles with other asanas.

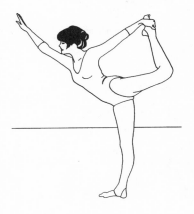

CHART YOUR PROGRESS - Degree of difficulty																	
	Hard						Easy			Hard							Easy
Date	1	2	3	4	5	6	7	8	Date	1	2	3	4	5	6	7	8

Chart Your Progress
Body Awareness

King of Dancer's Pose II

Date

_____

_____

_____

_____

_____

_____

_____

_____

_____

_____

_____

_____

_____

_____

_____

_____

_____

One-Leg Stand

(Eka Padasana)
(Eka, one; pada, leg)

Benefits
Aids in balance and concentration, and strengthens leg muscles.

Basic position
Stand straight with your feet together. Raise your arms over your head with your fingers together.

Instructions
Slowly lean forward, keeping your arms, head, and body in a straight line.
Simultaneously raise your right leg and stretch it backward.
Keep your leg in a straight line with the rest of your body.
Your body should rotate from the left hip joint.
The asana is attained when the arms, head, body, and right leg are in one straight horizontal line.
The left leg should be straight and vertical.
Remain in the posture for as long as you comfortably can.
Slowly return to the starting position.
Repeat the movement raising the left leg backward.
Repeat three times on each side.

Breathing
Inhale while raising the arms.
Exhale while assuming the final posture.
Breathe normally while in the posture.
Inhale while returning to the starting position.

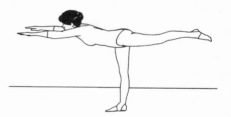

CHART YOUR PROGRESS - Degree of difficulty

Date	Hard 1	2	3	4	5	6	7	Easy 8	Date	Hard 1	2	3	4	5	6	7	Easy 8

Chart Your Progress
Body Awareness

One-Leg Stand

Date

Tree Pose

(Vrikshasana)
(Vriksha, tree)

Benefits

Tones and strengthens the legs, improves balance, stretches and tones the abdominal organs, and aids digestion.

Basic position

Stand with your feet together and your arms relaxed at your sides.
Be sure your weight is distributed evenly between the balls of your feet and your heels.

Instructions

Hold your head straight and focus your eyes on a specific point.
Place the sole of your right foot on the inside of your left thigh.
You may find it helpful to guide your foot into position with your right hand.
When your foot is in place and you feel you have your balance, slowly raise your arms above your head. Place your palms together and straighten your elbows.
Continue stretching upward as you hold the position.
Hold the posture as long as you comfortably can.
Slowly return to the original position.
Change legs and repeat.
Do the asana three times on each side.

Breathing

Inhale while establishing the position.
Breathe normally while in the posture.
Exhale while returning to the starting position.

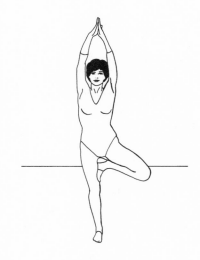

CHART YOUR PROGRESS - Degree of difficulty

	Hard						Easy			Hard						Easy
Date	1	2	3	4	5	6	7	8	Date	1	2	3	4	5	6	7	8

Chart Your Progress
Body Awareness

Tree Pose

Date

_____

_____

_____

_____

_____

_____

_____

_____

_____

_____

_____

_____

_____

_____

_____

_____

Half-Moon Pose
(Ardha Chandrasana)
(Ardha, half; chandra, moon)

Benefits
Stretches the arms and rib cage, and
when done on the toes, it firms the leg
muscles.

Basic position
While standing straight with your arms
over your head, interlace your fingers.

Instructions
Slowly bend from your waist as far as you
can stretch to your right side.
Slowly return to your original position.
Slowly bend to your left side.
Slowly return to your original position.
Try to balance on your toes every time
you do this asana. This way you will
slowly improve your sense of balance.
Bend five times to each side.

Breathing
Inhale as you stretch your arms over
your head.
Exhale as you bend to the side.
Inhale as you straighten up.

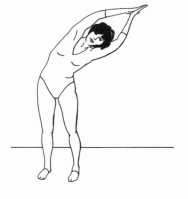

CHART YOUR PROGRESS - Degree of difficulty																	
	Hard						Easy			Hard							Easy
Date	1	2	3	4	5	6	7	8	Date	1	2	3	4	5	6	7	8

Chart Your Progress
Body Awareness

Half-Moon Pose

Date

_____

_____

_____

_____

_____

_____

_____

_____

_____

_____

_____

_____

_____

_____

_____

_____

Palm Tree Pose

(Talasana)
(**Tala**, palm tree)

Benefits
Strengthens the back, stomach, legs and feet, and helps develop balance and correct posture.

Basic position
Stand with your feet four to six inches apart and your arms comfortably at your sides.
Distribute the weight of your body evenly on both feet.

Instructions
Raise your arms over your head with your fingers reaching upward.
Look up at your hands.
Slowly rise up onto your toes and completely stretch your whole body.
Hold the asana as long as you wish.
Slowly return to your original position.
Repeat between three and five times.

Breathing
Inhale as you stretch up.
Hold your breath during your final stretch.
Exhale as you return to your original position.

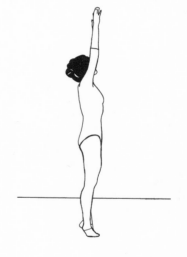

CHART YOUR PROGRESS - Degree of difficulty

	Hard							Easy		Hard							Easy
Date	1	2	3	4	5	6	7	8	Date	1	2	3	4	5	6	7	8

Chart Your Progress
Body Awareness

Palm Tree Pose

Date

The Peacock

(Mayurasana)
(Mayur, peacock)

Benefits
Strengthens the abdominal muscles, arms and shoulders, and is excellent for balance and coordination.

Basic position
Kneel on the floor with your feet together and your knees apart.
Place your palms flat on the floor between your knees with the fingers pointing toward your feet.

Instructions
In a kneeling position, bend your arms at the elbows so that the elbows point backward and are together at the abdomen.
Simultaneously lean forward and rest the abdomen on your upper arms and elbows.
Keeping your feet together, stretch your legs backward until they are straight.
Raise your head upward and rest the weight of your body on your hands and the tips of your toes (eventually you will be able to lift your toes).
Hold the asana for as long as you comfortably can and then slowly return to the basic position.
Each time you do the asana, attempt to increase the length of time you spend in the final position.

Breathing
Breathe normally throughout the exercise.

Limitations
Do not practice this asana if you have ulcers, hernia, high blood pressure, or an infection of any kind. This is one of the most difficult asanas and requires considerable practice.

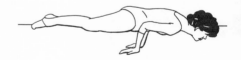

CHART YOUR PROGRESS - Degree of difficulty

	Hard						Easy		Hard						Easy
Date	1	2	3	4	5	6	7	8	Date	1	2	3	4	5	6	7	8

Chart Your Progress
Body Awareness

The Peacock

Date

_____

_____

_____

_____

_____

_____

_____

_____

_____

_____

_____

_____

_____

_____

_____

_____

_____

_____

_____

Insight
Further Your Self-Discovery

Many people have used the path of yoga as a means for continued growth and self-awareness. By reading one or more of the books listed below, you can gain many new insights and a further appreciation of the countless values of yoga.

Dass, Ram, **The Only Dance There Is**, New York, Anchor Books, 1974.

Fox, Emmett, **The Emmett Fox Treasury**, New York, Harper & Row, 1979.

Gandhi, Mohandas K., **An Autobiography**, Boston, Beacon Press, 1957.

Swami Muktananda, **Play of Consciousness**, San Francisco, Harper & Row, 1978.

Yogananda, Paramahansa, **Autobiography of a Yogi**, Los Angeles, Self-Realization Fellowship Publishers, 1971.

Bibliography

Dass, Ram, **The Only Dance There Is**, New York, Anchor Books, 1974.

Gandhi, Mohandas K., **An Autobiography**, Boston, Beacon Press, 1957.

Hathaway, Monica Lind, and Hathaway, Harmon, **Yoga for Athletics**, Chicago, Contemporary Books, 1978.

Hittleman, Richard, **Yoga 28 Day Exercise Plan**, New York, Workman Publishing Co., 1969.

Iyengar, B.K.S., **The Concise Light on Yoga**, New York, Schocken Books, 1982.

Kent, Howard, **A Color Guide to Yoga**, Secaucus, NJ, Chartwell Books, 1980.

Kirschner, M.J., **Yoga all Your Life**, New York, Schocken Books, 1982.

Lidell, Lucy, **The Sivananda Companion to Yoga**, New York, Simon & Schuster, 1987.

Smith, Bob, and Smith, Linda Bourderau, **Yoga for a New Age**, Seattle, WA, Smith Productions, 1986.

Taylor, Louise, and Bryant, Betty, **Acupressure Yoga and You**, Tokyo and New York, Japan Publications, 1984.

Taylor, Louise, and Bryant, Betty, **Ki: Energy For Everybody**, Tokyo and New York, Japan Publications, 1990.

Yogananda, Paramahansa, **Autobiography of a Yogi**, Los Angeles, Self-Realization Fellowship, 1971.

About the Author

Louise Taylor received her master of science degree from California State University, Northridge. Her studies of hatha yoga took her to India, where she had a first hand impression of the yogic system. She is a student of Siddha Yoga, and as a devotee of Guru Swami Chidvilasananda, she has practiced yogic disciplines for the past ten years. Ms. Taylor has taught health-oriented courses at Mount Saint Mary's College in Los Angeles, at Los Angeles Mission College, California State University, Northridge, and at Santa Monica College. In 1984 she founded the Healing Arts Center in Woodland Hills, California, and currently directs this Center, which teaches a variety of alternative health practices including many aspects of yoga.

Ms. Taylor is a co-author of **Acupressure, Yoga, and You**, which integrates the benefits of hatha yoga and acupressure; and **Ki: Energy for Everybody,** a look at ways to improve the body and increase your energy from both the Eastern and Western perspectives. She also has developed a cassette tape, **Color Meditations: for Adults and Children,** which guides its listeners into peaceful, stress-free meditations as well as balancing the powerful **chakra** energy centers.

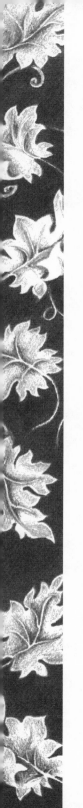

Your Journal